TWIN RESEARCH

Part A

Psychology and Methodology

PROGRESS IN CLINICAL AND BIOLOGICAL RESEARCH

Series Editors
George J. Brewer
Vincent P. Eijsvoogel

Robert Grover
Kurt Hirschhorn
Seymour S. Kety

Sidney Undenfriend
Jonathan W. Uhr

TWIN RESEARCH

Proceedings of the Second International
Congress on Twin Studies
August 29—September 1, 1977
Washington, DC

Part A
Psychology and Methodology

EDITOR

WALTER E NANCE
Chairman, Department of Human Genetics
Virginia Commonwealth University
Medical College of Virginia
Richmond, Virginia

ASSOCIATE EDITORS

GORDON ALLEN
National Institute of Mental Health
Rockville, Maryland

and

PAOLO PARISI
Gregor Mendel Institute
Rome, Italy

ALAN R LISS, INC • NEW YORK • 1978

© 1978 Alan R. Liss, Inc.

Address all inquiries to the publisher:

Alan R. Liss, Inc.
150 Fifth Avenue
New York, New York 10011

Printed in the United States of America

Library of Congress Cataloging in Publication Data

International Congress on Twin Studies, 2d,
      Washington, D.C., 1977.
      Twin research.

      (Progress in clinical and biological research;
v. 24, pts. A—C)
      Includes bibliographies.
      Contents: pt. A. Psychology and methodology. — pt. B.
Biology and epidemiology. — pt. C. Clinical studies.
      1. Twins — Congresses. 2. Twins — Psychology —
Congresses. 3. Diseases in twins — Congresses.
4. Birth, Multiple — Congresses. I. Nance, Walter E.
II. Allen, Gordon, 1919—
III. Parisi, Paolo. IV. Title. V. Series
[DNLM: 1. Twins — Congresses. 2. Research —
Congresses. W1 PR668E v. 24 / WQ235 I59 1977t]
RG696.I55   1977   618.2'5   78-8480

3 Volume Set ISBN 0-08451-0024-6
Part A: Psychology and Methodology ISBN 0-8451-0150-1

Contributors

A Bertelsen, Institute of Psychiatric Demography, Psychiatric Hospital, Aarhus, Denmark **119**

Kathryn Norcross Black, Department of Psychological Sciences, Purdue University, Lafayette, IN 47907 **145**

R Darrell Bock, Departments of Science and Education, University of Chicago, Chicago, IL 60637 **211**

CE Boklage, Department of Biostatistics and the Genetics Curriculum, The University of North Carolina, Chapel Hill, NC 27514 **189**

Joe C Christian, Department of Medical Genetics, Indiana University School of Medicine, Indiana University Medical Center, Indianapolis, IN 46202 **145**

Donald J Cohen, Child Study Center and Departments of Psychiatry and Pediatrics, Yale University, New Haven, CT 06520 **245**

Linda A Corey, Department of Human Genetics, Medical College of Virginia, Richmond, VA 23298 **201**

E Defrise-Gussenhoven, Professor of the Free University of Brussels, Centrum for Statistics and Laboratory for Human Genetics, 2 Pleinlaan, Brussel 1050 Belgium **237**

David L Demets, Biometrics Research Branch, National Heart, Lung, and Blood Institute, National Institutes of Health, Bethesda, MD 20014 **253**

Eleanor Dibble, National Institute of Mental Health, Bethesda, MD 20014 **245**

Robert H Dworkin, Department of Psychology, Cornell University, Ithaca, NY 14853 **49**

LJ Eaves, Genetics Department, University of Birmingham, England **152**

RC Elston, Department of Biostatistics and the Genetics Curriculum, The University of North Carolina, Chapel Hill, NC 27514 **189**

Richard R Fabsitz, Epidemiology Branch, National Heart, Lung, and Blood Institute, National Institutes of Health, Bethesda, MD 20014 **253**

U de Faire, Department of Medicine, Serafimerlasarettet, S-112 83 Stockholm, Sweden **63**

Manning Feinleib, Epidemiology Branch, National Heart, Lung, and Blood Institute, National Institutes of Health, Bethesda, MD 20014 **253**

Brain D Sank Firschein, Rockland Research Institute, Orangeburg, NY 10962 **137**

Siv Fischbein, Department of Educational Research, School of Education, Stockholm, Sweden **101**

The boldface number following each participants' name is the opening page number of that author's paper.

Jo Anne Frohock, Department of Graduate Art Therapy, Pratt Institute, Brooklyn, NY 11205 **35**

DW Fulker, Department of Psychology, Institute of Psychiatry, The Bethlem Royal Hospital, Beckenham, Kent BR3 3BX England **217**

Josef E Garai, Department of Graduate Art Therapy, Pratt Institute, Brooklyn, NY 11205 **35**

Arleen S Garfinkle, Institute for Behavioral Genetics, University of Colorado, Boulder, CO 80309 **95**

Robert J Garrison, Epidemiology Branch, National Heart, Lung, and Blood Institute, National Institutes of Health, Bethesda, MD 20014 **253**

Edward Grant, Department of Psychology, College of Cape Breton, Sydney, Nova Scotia B1P 6K3 Canada **111**

Jane M Grawe, Child Study Center and Departments of Psychiatry and Pediatrics, Yale University, New Haven, CT 06520 **245**

Einar Kringlen, Institute of Behavioral Sciences in Medicine, University of Oslo, Preklinisk Medisin, Sognsvannv 9, Oslo 3, Norway **131**

Allan R Kuse, Institute for Behavioral Genetics, University of Colorado, Boulder, CO 80302 **25**

John C Loehlin, Psychology Department, University of Texas, Austin, TX 78712 **69**

Hugh Lytton, Department of Educational Psychology, University of Calgary, Calgary, Alberta T2N 1N4 Canada **43**

NG Martin, Department of Genetics, University of Birmingham, Birmingham B15 2TT England **13**

Walter E Nance, Department of Human Genetics, Medical College of Virginia, Richmond, VA 23298 **201**

Diane Sank, Rockland Research Center, Orangeburg, New York, and City College, City University of New York, New York, NY 10031 **137**

Alan Searleman, Department of Psychology, State University of New York, Stony Brook, NY 11790 **57**

James Shields, Department of Psychiatry, Institute of Psychiatry (Genetics Section), De Crespigny Park, London SE5 8AF England **79**

Sally P Springer, Department of Psychology, State University of New York, Stony Brook, NY 11790 **57**

C Susanne, Professor for the Free University of Brussels, Centrum for Statistics and Laboratory for Human Genetics, 2 Pleinlaan, Brussel 1050, Belgium **237**

Paul Taubman, Department of Economics, University of Pennsylvania, Philadelphia, PA 19104 **175**

T Theorell, Department of Medicine, Serafimerlasarettet, S-112 83 Stockholm, Sweden **63**

Svenn Torgersen, Institute of Behavioral Sciences in Medicine, University of Oslo, Preklinisk Medisin, Sognsvannv 9, Oslo 3, Norway **125**

Steven G Vandenberg, Institute for Behavioral Genetics, University of Colorado, Boulder, CO 80302 **25, 95**

Patricia Welch, Department of Psychological Sciences, Purdue University, Lafayette, IN 47907 **145**

René Zazzo, Laboratory of Child Psychology (Ecole Pratique des Hautes Etudes) 75005 Paris, France **1**

Preface

Since Galton introduced the twin study method in 1876, this technique and modifications of it have been widely used as an approach to solving the nature-nurture question. Over the years, as knowledge about the epidemiology, biology, and psychology of twins has accumulated, an increasingly complete understanding of both the power and limitations of twin methodology has emerged. Novel approaches such as the study of monozygotic twins reared apart, co-twin control studies, multivariate analyses of twin data, and the monozygotic twin half-sib study design, as well as the classical twin model, constitute some of the most incisive methods available for clinical trials as well as for the analysis of both quantitative and qualitative traits in man.

These three volumes on "Psychology and Methodology," "Epidemiology and Biology," and "Clinical Studies" include both invited and contributed papers that were presented at the Second International Congress on Twin Studies which was held in Washington, DC, from August 29 to September 1, 1977. The Congress was sponsored by the International Society for Twin Studies and the number, quality, and diversity of the papers included in these volumes attests to the resurgence of interest in research for the benefit of twins that has occurred since the Society was founded in 1974.

The organizers of the Congress are particularly grateful to the National Institute of Child Health and Human Development for its support of the Congress under Grant #HD 10663–01.

Walter E Nance, MD, PhD
Richmond, Virginia
May, 1978

Contents

Genesis and Peculiarities of the Personality of Twins

René Zazzo

To speak of the personality of twins, and to assume, by that, that their personality presents traits that are strictly their own, is to abandon the postulates of the classical twin method, established 100 years ago by Francis Galton and still practiced today, continually refined and continually questioned, in the analysis of the powers of heredity.

Galton's first postulate, barely formulated because of its immediate evidence for any researcher, is that twins, both identical and fraternal, have nothing which differentiates them from singletons. This postulate appears to be an absolute prerequisite of the twin method. To prove the powers of heredity and to serve as a source of universal evidence, twins would have to be like everybody else.

In fact, no one has ever seriously doubted that twins should be genetically similar to nontwins: There is no reason why they would not inherit traits like anyone else and under the same conditions common to our species.

But this postulate about twins being similar to nontwins does not only involve heredity, since the powers of heredity are not evaluated per se but in relation to other influences — those of the environment.

It is therefore necessary to admit that the relationship of heredity and environment is the same with twins and nontwins alike. That is to say, the environment within which twins live and develop is no different from that of the rest of mankind.

Now, it is on this point that doubt is permitted, that the twin method is subject to caution. Should the above statement prove incorrect, we would doubtless lose a method, but we would win a new object of research: a special personality for twins.

On admitting the peculiarities of the twin environment, one would quasi-necessarily conclude that there is a twin psychism. We will soon come back to that.

Twin Research: Psychology and Methodology, pages 1–11

But there is first reason to question the blindness of authors to this problem of environment. True, and we have already said it, environmental factors, as well as hereditary factors, should present no peculiarity in twins for them to provide universal evidence. Nevertheless, one should not believe that the first authors, and Galton [1875] in the first place, have treated the problem with any constraint. For them, the problem does not exist. Some 50 years passed until 1937 when Newman, Freeman, and Holzinger published their book, "Twins, A Study of Heredity and Environment," before the problem appeared, but at that point the authors very easily attempted to minimize or deny it.

If the problem of a twin environment did not exist in Galton's time, it is largely because the very notion of environment was hardly a problem. Environment is nurture as opposed to nature; it is the whole of the physical and cultural nourishment with which the individual is formed and sustains himself. Starting with such a broad and vague definition, it would hardly occur to anyone that the environment where twins live may be any different from that of singletons, or that the environment of identical twins may be any different from that of fraternal twins, and less still (and I insist on stressing this last proposition) *that the two twin partners of one and the same couple, when more closely examined, may appear to live in two different environments.* It is, in effect, this last proposition, the most unthinkable of all and that which justifies all other ones, that will break down the classical paradigm of the twin method.

This proposition first of all suggests a hypothesis, doubtless the only one that may account for a paradoxical fact: Identical twins are not psychologically identical, even though they are raised together. Hence, they have the same heredity and same environment (in the usual sense of the word) and nevertheless, different personalities. Where, then, does the difference come from?

My answer is known, as I proposed it more than 20 years ago: *The difference is a couple effect.*

Such a couple effect requires one to refine and revise the notion of environment, and maybe even get rid of it, for the benefit of a more analytical and pertinent conception.

Why have the facts not implied this hypothesis earlier? One only sees, it is said, what one looks for, that which corresponds to a necessarily partial reading grid. That is not entirely true. The grid also lets unexpected phenomena pass. And one perceives them, but does one's best to consider them meaningless and absorb them in the inherent margin of error of all observations and measures. Thus, the difference that one observes in the scores of two co-twins on a personality test is easy to account for, upon invoking at the same time the intraindividual fluctuations of each partner and the gross lack of sensibility of the test.

But then comes a day when the accumulation of contradictions is no longer acceptable and a threshold of nontolerance is attained. Then the reading grid breaks, and a new view asserts itself. In any case, this is what has happened to me during my twin studies. Those twin partners that I had until then regarded as identical beings suddenly appeared to me as distinct and dissimilar. A total reversal in perspective occurred, and everything was again brought to question. The new "whys" arose.

On the other hand, it is likely that the accumulation of contradictions alone may not cause such a conversion. Favorable occasions are implied, as well as an evolution of ideas and sensibilities concerning all of psychology.

If the differences between co-twins failed to appear earlier, this is partly because the traits in which researchers were interested actually were hardly different and influenced by the couple effect little or not at all. The emphasis was then on the cognitive functions: scholastic output, mnemonic and perceptive aptitudes and, of course, the famous intelligence quotient.

It was with the increasing development of the so-called personality tests that the differences eventually appeared, that the contradictions to the dogma of identity accumulated. But the lack of objectivity of these tests has served for a long time as an argument to doubt these differences.

At the same time of the expanded usage of these tests, the primary importance of the notion of personality asserted itself among psychologists, together with the idea, until then held very discreetly and apprehensively, that the personality of each is formed in his relationship with others, that the we is anterior to the I and determines it.

In the course of my works, which resulted in the 1960 publication "Les jumeaux: le couple et la personne" ("Twins, the Couple and the Person"), it is quite evident that all these factors played a role, factors both of general nature and stemming from my personal experience, in shaping the notion of couple effect. I no longer view twins as a double, as the same being in two copies, but as a couple. And that is why I prefer the expression "couple" to that of "pair."

Now, the couple situation excludes the identicalness of the partners, the same as a dialogue excludes two parallel discourses. A couple unconsciously or consciously implies diversity, complementarity or opposition or alternation, in functions and roles. It is in the logic of the couple and its structure to create interdependent and different beings — different because of their interdependence. Their difference is a couple effect.

The simplest illustration of the structure of the couple is its relation of dominance or leadership. Such a relation may almost always be observed in monozygotic (MZ) as well as in dizygotic (DZ) couples, although in a rather variable way. The relationship established since prime infancy may reverse itself with age, or even at the same age, as a result of tasks and situations. One of the twins may have to deal with the outer world, whereas the co-twin takes care of the couple's private life. This is what Helmut von Bracken has referred to in terms of Minister of Foreign Affairs and Minister of the Interior. And it is not infrequent that one of the twins plays both roles.

All laws, however, have their degrees of application. Under what conditions and for what reasons is the law of dominance applied to the benefit of one twin rather than his co-twin.

Upon researching all that could be related to very early observable dominance, I made a number of very diverse observations. Dominance may result from higher birthweight or better physical conditions, or even from having been designated and then treated as the elder twin, whatever the criteria the parents follow in so doing. It is indeed amusing to see that 50% of the parents consider as elder the first born, and 50% the second born. What is important, however, is to be considered as such. The dominance in the twin couple can also be established in response to the dominance in the parental couple: Each of the twins is taken by each of the parents and more or less shaped to the parent's image.

It is difficult to know if one of these factors alone, of these cause-pretexts, could suffice to orient the relation of dominance, but it clearly appears that the whole of them is decisive.

We end up, at any rate, at a question which is at the same time one of terminology and of method: The minor inequalities observable at birth and the couple effects are obviously not of a hereditary nature; should we therefore classify them under "environment" or should we develop a third term for them? I would tend to reject the term of environment, which is, for psychologists, too narrowly associated with the idea of "sociocultural." If it is useful to have one universal term to contrast with "heredity," why not simply speak of "nongenetic factors?" The diversity of these factors and their respective roles should then be analyzed, and this is the essential thing. The couple effect is one of these factors: a factor so far ignored because of the tenacious and blinding bipolar notion, heredity versus environment, that proposed, in other words, the opposition of two entities, the individual in his solitude and the environment.

The couple does not exist, except in a secondary and contingent way. It is devoid of all effectiveness, of all scientific stature. It is only good for private life and for novels. Otherwise, how could it be explained that psychologists have studied twin couples for so long without ever taking into account that they are couples?

The slow germination of the couple concept in the scientific world makes me think of Gregor Mendel's study of peas. May this concept eventually have the same success!

Let us not speak of France. The psychologists of my country, blocked by the phobia of heredity, do not like to listen to talk about twins. And the only tangible result of my work would be to have inspired a celebrated novelist with a baroque and fantastic tale.

In Galton's country, on the other hand, the message has been heard, but at first received with circumspection. These concepts of twin situation, of couple effect, are interesting, they say, but supported by too little evidence, so that they still remain very speculative.

Peter Mittler's book "The Study of Twins," published in 1971, is very revealing of such an interest and reservation. In his preface, the author tells us that my work helped to orient him towards the field of twin studies. But then, in spite of this original orientation, the research studies he carries out (ie, the twin analysis of linguistic functions) eventually bring him back to the use of the classical twin method. The new notions are accepted by Mittler, and without a doubt by many other authors, but they fail to use them towards a "new deal" for twins because of a lack of a satisfactory formalization. For 100 years researchers have played with the formula of the relative roles of heredity versus environment and then, without giving up this solid tradition, they have worked out more or less sophisticated calculations for the evaluation of heredity. Other steps, other devices of comparison, other calculations, should now be imagined. And it is not that simple. Mittler's conclusions are in fact very explicit in this respect: "More information on the individuality and mutual relationship of the twin pair might well lead to a modification of design in twin studies of the future." (p 159).

This future will announce itself soon. Information multiplies, gradually imposes a new viewpoint, and eventually brings about a modification of the twin paradigm.

Among the most recent findings, the richest piece of information comes from a British researcher, Sandra Canter, an associate of Gordon Claridge at the Glasgow Department of Psychological Medicine.

The most surprising of all the fascinating results obtained by Sandra Canter concerns the trait of extroversion of the Eysenck Personality Inventory. The intraclass correlation coefficient is 0.67 in MZ twins living apart, and only 0.10, practically nil, in those living together.

In other words, genetic factors appear to play a very significant role when the twins live apart, but almost completely disappear when the twins live together.

Twins resemble each other less, or even not at all, when they live together. Same heredity, same environment, and yet no resemblance: There is the paradox.

This paradox sheds a new light on the process of personality development if one forgets about the classical formula, heredity versus environment. For this group of subjects and for the trait extroversion, the twin situation apparently erases genetic effects.

Of course, the role of the couple effect is not always as evident, not always as massive. It remains to be known in what cases it plays a role and with what relative force does it affect other categories and factors. That is exactly the problem of a new twin method, of a new formalization.

Thus, identical twins are not psychologically identical. This is the first piece of evidence I wanted to stress, a piece of evidence that implies a revision of the notion of environment and the recourse to the complementary notions of twin situation and of couple effect.

Still, once this is admitted, it would not necessarily follow that twins have a

personality of their own that would distinguish them from nontwins. The hypothesis is likely, but it should still be supported by facts.

But in what direction and with what criteria would one research the facts? In
short, how would one define, and then grasp, what is designated by the term,
personality? The answer to the problem of an originality of twins depends on
such a preliminary definition.

One could look for such an originality at the level of isolated mental traits, or
at the level of a general pattern, since personality is usually defined as the inte-
gration of physical and mental traits.

Whether we deal with isolated traits or with a pattern, a second question, however, arises: Does the assumed originality refer to all twins (all MZ twins, or even
all MZ and DZ twins, and for the latter, whether of like or unlike sex), or is it but
an *average truth,* ie, referred to twins as a group but not to each individual twin?
This is a very important question which, at a time when it is very fashionable to
refer to the problems of heredity, may refer to any human group, of racial,
ethnic, or social nature. To ask whether a twin personality exists is a question as
laden with ambiguities as to ask whether a Jewish personality, or a working-
class personality, exists.

I have to admit that I can give a precise answer only with respect to given
isolated traits and only from the viewpoint of average truths. Let me first look
at cognitive traits.

Based on an investigation carried out on a sample of about 100,000 French
students, I could already show that the twin population is characterized by a
slightly lower intellectual development, as measured by a collective test like the
Binet-Simon. The result is practically overlapping in the seven socioeconomic
groups considered. Thus, in the lowest group, twins have an average IQ of 87, against
a general average of 93, whereas in the highest group twins have an IQ of 112
against a general IQ of 120. For the total population, the age range of which is
6–12 years, the average IQ in twins is 93. It should be noted, however, that in
unlike-sexed DZ pairs, the average IQ is only slightly lower than that of singletons
at an age of 6 years, and then catches up with the norm by an age of 12 years.

Aiming at finding out the genesis and components of this mental inferiority,
my colleague Irène Lézine and I have examined a sample of 28 twins (4 MZ and
10 DZ pairs) 1–4 years old. The Developmental Quotient, obtained by way of
Gesell's baby test, averaged 88. But much more interesting were the partial
quotients calculated for four sectors of development: Language development
was 75, social relations 65, whereas completely normal values were found for
postural development (100) and motor performance (100). This pattern was
found in all MZ and in most (8 out of 10) DZ pairs.

The normal values found for postural development and motor performance
show the twins studied to be free from any neurological deficit. The retardation
evaluated by the global IQ of 88 is thus entirely explained by the insufficient

development of those sectors where exchanges with the environment are involved: language and social relations.

Some recent observations, published by two of my collaborators [Richon and Plee, 1976], now bring new support to my old research, on which they perhaps also shed new light. In twins of school age examined with the Weschler Intelligent Scale for Children (WISC), the score for "performance" appears to be remarkably higher than the score for "verbal." This results in a much lower value than the norm of 100, whereas the value is higher than the norm of 100 in those tests where the role of language is apparently absent. The hypothesis of a process of compensation has thus been suggested.

Evidence of the same order is brought by the works of Koch [1966] and of Record et al. [1970].

Koch has administered Thurstone's Primary Mental Abilities Test, which allows for an analysis of different cognitive aptitudes, to a sample of 96 twin pairs 5–6 years old. Among other interesting results, he has observed, in all groups of twins, MZ and DZ, male and female alike, higher scores for perception tests and lower scores for tests where the verbal factor plays a role, with respect to the average values in nontwins. Lowest on verbal tests are the MZ twins' scores.

A much different study has been carried out by Record et al. [1970] who investigated the results of scholastic examinations for more than 50,000 adolescents. The 2,164 twins included in this population had an average score of 95.7 for tests on verbal reasoning, whereas nontwins scored 100.1. But an extremely interesting result was obtained, an absolutely new one in the twin literature: Out of the total 2,164, the 148 twins that had lost their twin partner, deceased at birth or in early infancy, scored very close to the nontwin average, 98.8. Now, these 148 surviving twins had a birthweight comparable, on the average, to that of their deceased co-twins, so that it can be excluded that physiological factors should, at least totally, account for the lower scores on verbal aptitudes.

Last, but not least, a much more detailed analysis has been carried out by Peter Mittler [1972] on verbal aptitudes in twins and the respective role of genetic versus environmental factors in the determination of their lower scores. Once more, in this research carried out with the Illinois Test of Psycholinguistic Abilities (ITPA), what first appears is a global inferiority in language development. The 200 twins, exactly 4 years old, show an average delay of six months with respect to a control sample of 100 nontwins. No significant difference between MZ and DZ twins is found.

But the utilization of the ITPA, with its nine subtests which correspond to nine aspects of linguistic behavior, allows better understanding of how this global result is obtained.

Starting with the classical comparison between MZ and DZ twins, it is noted that the difference between MZ correlations and DZ correlations varies considerably from one subtest to another. This suggests that the relative influences of heredity and environment are not uniform for all linguistic aspects: audiovocal tests, ie, those in which the child actually has to speak, are the most environmentally influenced, whereas visual-motor tests are the most genetically influenced. Here one perhaps recovers the contrast between the perceptive factor and the verbal factor as stressed in Koch's research.

Once these results were obtained with the twin comparison, Mittler carried out a comparison among sociocultural strata with the control sample of 100 nontwins. The results confirmed those obtained in the former survey: The environmental difference is reflected in a difference of linguistic performance at all levels, but the audiovocal abilities are those that account the most for the verbal inferiority of the children belonging to lower sociocultural strata.

All of these works, covering a diversity of populations and techniques, finally outline a very coherent general picture. In the very wide range of ages considered, from 1 year through adolescence, twins are characterized, on the average, by a slightly lower intellectual development as a whole. This is mostly, if not totally, due to a linguistic deficit; more precisely, to a linguistic deficit at the level of its oral expression. It is possible that this deficit is compensated for, to some extent and for some twins, by the higher development of other functions, perceptive and manipulative in nature. These characteristics may be observed in both classes of twins, but more clearly in MZ twins. Pre- and perinatal factors (troubles of pregnancy and of delivery, prematurity, small weight) may only slightly account, if they do, for the linguistic deficit.

All of the cited authors thus end up by attributing this deficit to a postnatal factor: the twin situation.

True, the notion of a language retardation in twins is not new: It had already been noted by the beginning of the century. What is really new is the hypothesis of a postnatal factor; what is absolutely recent is the analysis of this retardation and the accumulation of evidence supporting this hypothesis.

The effects of the twin situation, as analyzed through tests, may be grasped at the origin through the direct observation of strange behavior in twins at the very beginning of language development: This is what the Russian psychologist Luria identifies as *autonomous language* [Luria and Youdovitch, 1959], meaning by that an archaic language, making use of sounds, words, and syntax that are not those of the common language and that I myself identify as *cryptophasia,* in order to stress its incommunicability to others [Zazzo, 1949, 1960].

Much before its utilization in play or for specific secrecy reasons, the autonomous language means first of all that the twins can suffice to themselves. The twin situation is the limit value, the extreme case of any couple situation. Of all that we can imagine on the couple dialectic, self-assertion and permanent risk of alienation, and of all that we can divine about the powers and consequences of our relations with others, identical twins offer us the best possible analysis.

The life of a couple has therefore contradictory effects. It differentiates and yet makes uniform; it confers to genetically identical partners dissimilarities that cannot be ascribed to environmental forces, as well as similarities that cannot be ascribed to heredity.

And so it is with cryptophasia — at the same time a specific characteristic of twins and a factor of inferiority. What roles does this trait, relative to language development, play in what might be the personality of twins?

We do not know very much about this hypothetical personality. Legends, popular traditions, and romantic literature have always attributed unusual traits to twins. And now parapsychology ascribes them exceptional gifts. But our scientific evidence is extremely scanty, and this is not because of experimental difficulties, but because twins have always served psychology, whereas psychology has almost never served twins.

Nevertheless, both through the situation from which it arises and through its effects, cryptophasia may serve as a solid thread that one can pull in an attempt to unroll the complex skein of personality, somewhat like Cuvier who, with a fragment of a fossil, brought about the reconstruction of an unknown species. However, in our case we are not dealing with a law of harmony of forms but with a chain of causes and effects.

It is not possible that the way in which most of the twins enter the world of language has no effect on the orientation of their development, on the construction of the pattern that becomes known as personality. We already know that cryptophasia results in a retardation of socialized language, affects conceptualization, and may also originate overcompensations. One has to go deeper. Language is not only an instrument of expression and communication; while internalizing, it also becomes an instrument of regulation for our thoughts and acts.

Whereas in some perceptive or manipulatory tests twins score close to, or even higher than, the norm, they appear to score lower on other tasks that are also nonverbal, but require a capacity for organization, foresight, and planning. That is the paradoxical picture presented by the twins examined in our laboratory: In spite of their relatively brilliant results on the WISC, they accumulate errors in tests like Porteus mazes, where the subject must constantly regulate his activity. All kinds of supporting strategies then appear, including aloud verbalization, thus showing the need for and lack of internal language. The twins also behave in a childish and impulsive way on the Rorschach test. And it should be noted that this picture is common to the twins we studied and to other subjects who are similarly affected by a remarkable retardation in language development [Richon and Plee, 1976]. Language retardation may therefore have long-term consequences that far exceed the cognitive domain.

One should hypothesize that the situation responsible for cryptophasia and for language retardation continues, at other levels and in different ways, to exert its influence.

I will not refer again to my previous studies on the "shyness" of twins, or on the subject of marriage, where couple effects are clearly evident: One could discuss endlessly their choice of the partner, conjugal difficulties, or intratwin marriages. One point deserves special consideration, however, and this is the abnormal rate of the single state: In a survey I have carried out, through the registry of one district of Paris, on all twins born over a period of 20 years (1883–1902), the single state has appeared to be 50% higher in the twin population than in the general population.

No indication whatsoever is found in the literature concerning the characteristics of twins in terms of sociability and emotional behavior. Sandra Canter's recent work [Canter, 1973] is a very good indication in this respect. She has administered four tasks to twins, covering a total of about 30 personality traits or factors. She has reported all intraclass correlations for the twins of all groups, separated and nonseparated, MZ and DZ. But she has failed to report the scores themselves! Clearly, she is interested in the twin situation as a factor that may alter the balance between heredity and environment, but not at all *in the twins as individuals.* And yet, her article is entitled, "Personality traits in twins."

These traits will certainly be uncovered in the years to come. The question is now posed, and it cannot remain without an answer. For twins, it is also just that, after having served psychology for so long, psychology should serve them in turn. Today, all that is known about twins appears to be negative: retarded mental development, retarded language development, lower sociability. A more attentive and better oriented study will possibly reveal positive traits and unrecognized capabilities. Educators will then be able to differentiate those couple effects that should be cultivated from those that should be neutralized.

This twin psychology that we have caught a glimpse of today has, as its object, 2% of the population. This is already not negligible. But, as a matter of fact, it concerns all of us.

To arrive at this conclusion, one must avoid the error of locking twins in their twinhood. This is a type of error that depends on our lack of mental flexibility. When we have to understand any particular group of individuals, either we try to assimilate them to the general population, or we throw them back into the ghetto of their own peculiarity.

The peculiarities of twins, like any other peculiarities of a social, ethnic, or biological order, are probably nothing more than the marked expression of traits that we all possess to different degrees. Because of its perfection and effects, the couple serves as a screen for the surrounding world; it limits the richness of verbal exchange with adults; it restrains the acquisition of socialized and conceptual forms of language, favoring purely emotional and "synpractical" ones, ie, forms closely connected to the ongoing activity.

Whereas in any couple by choice or chance the creations of the common life are inextricably mixed with the initial differences of the partners, in the case of identical twins everything begins with zero and in complete equality of biological blueprint.

Twins, and only twins, can allow us to understand the diversity of couple effects upon the diversity of mental traits, and to understand how an individuality is formed, an individuality in its relations with others.

According to the classic approach, data derived from twin studies have no general value unless the peculiarities of twins are denied. In our new perspective, it is precisely their peculiarities that give us information on the most complex processes of our personality. We may thus start, at the same time, with a twin psychology and our own psychology.

And thus, it seems to me that we can realize the so far impossible dream of Arnold Gesell, who first originated my passionate interest in twins. According to him, the singleton is frequently a twin who is unaware of being such, or an incomplete twin: unaware twin, if the partner disappeared, totally reabsorbed in the course of gestation; incomplete twin, much more frequently, through the phenomenon of hemihypertrophy, the asymmetry between right and left parts of the body being the beginning of a twinning process.

My own point today is less ambitious, since it does not refer to embryology, but is much more general, concerning the genesis of any personality. Psychologically and to different degrees, we are all twins.

REFERENCES

Canter S (1973): Personality traits in twins. In Claridge G (ed): "Personality Differences and Biological Variations. A Study of Twins." Oxford: Pergamon Press.

Galton F (1875): The history of twins as a criterion of the relative powers of nature and nurture. Fraser's Magazine, 12:566–576.

Koch HL (1966): "Twins and Twin Relations." Chicago: University of Chicago Press.

Luria AR, Youdovitch FJ (1959): "Speech and Development of Mental Processes in the Child." London: Staples Press. [Originally published in Russian: Moscow: Acad Pedag Sci RSFSR, (1956)].

Mittler P (1971): "The Study of Twins." Penguin Books.

Mittler P (1972): Genetic and environmental influences on language abilities. (In French). Enfance 5:519–530.

Newman HH, Freeman FN, Holzinger KJ (1937): "Twins: A Study of Heredity and Environment." Chicago: University of Chicago Press.

Record RG, McKeown T, Edwards JH (1970): An investigation of the difference in measured intelligence between twins and single births. Ann Hum Genet 34:11–20.

Richon G, Plee B (1976): A propos de la dichotomie verbal/non verbal. Enfance 4–5:495–509.

Zazzo R (1949): Cryptophasie et situation gémellaire. Congrès Pédiatres de langue française, Actes 308–312. Paris: Expansion Scientifique Francaise.

Zazzo R (1960): "Les jumeaux: le couple et la personne." Presses Universitaires de France.

Genetics of Sexual and Social Attitudes in Twins

NG Martin

While most social scientists have adjusted to the idea that variation in cognitive abilities has a genetic component, many would regard it as improbable that such allegedly malleable traits as attitudes to social or sexual questions could be influenced by genetic differences between individuals. Most would guess that social forces and cultural inheritance were more potent molders of individual differences in political opinions. A simple screening test for the relative importance of these sources of variation is provided by the classical study of monozygotic (MZ) and dizygotic (DZ) twins reared together.

THE DATA

The results from three different twin studies are summarized in this paper. The three twin samples were obtained at intervals of two to three years by postal questionnaire from the Maudsley Twin Register maintained at the Institute of Psychiatry, London, by Professor HJ Eysenck and Mrs J Kasriel. The register consists of volunteer twins, 18—56 years old at the time of sampling, obtained through appeals in the media, and makes no claim to either randomness or representativeness. Nevertheless most pertinent sample means and variances do not differ markedly from those found in carefully randomized samples. Zygosity was ascertained largely by postal questionnaire, the reliability of which was checked by blood grouping a subsample of the twins. The question of zygosity diagnosis in the Maudsley Twin Register is discussed fully in Kasriel and Eaves [1976]. The breakdown of the three samples by zygosity and sex can be seen in Table III.

Study I obtained responses of 823 twin pairs to an early 68-item version of the Eysenck Public Opinion Inventory. This was scored for the two principal factors extracted — a Radical vs Conservative dimension and a Tough- vs

Twin Research: Psychology and Methodology, pages 13—23

Tenderminded dimension. Preliminary results of genetical analysis of this survey have been reported by Eaves and Eysenck [1974] and more extensively by Hewitt [1974].

Study II was an anonymous survey whose principal aim was to obtain responses to Eysenck's Sexual Attitudes Questionnaire [Eysenck, 1976]. Because of the nature of the survey, only 246 pairs responded. Two main attitudes factors were extracted and labeled "Sexual Satisfaction" and "Libido." In addition, responses to a more recent 88-item version of the Public Opinion Inventory were obtained and scored for factors Radicalism and Toughmindedness. Results of this study have been discussed fully in Martin [1977] and published in Martin and Eysenck [1976] and Martin et al [1977].

Study III used a quite different questionnaire, the Wilson-Patterson Conservatism Scale [Wilson, 1973], and obtained factor scores on the Radicalism dimension for 587 twin pairs. No factor equivalent to Eysenck's "Toughmindedness" could be extracted. The results of this study are discussed fully in Last [in preparation] and the joint results and conclusions of all three studies will be published by Eaves et al [in preparation].

THE ANALYSIS AND ITS POWER

The biometrical genetic approach to the analysis of twin data has now been discussed extensively in the literature [eg, Eaves and Eysenck, 1975; Martin, 1975]. Briefly, after the data have been rescaled to remove scale-dependent genotype-environment interaction (detected by the regression of MZ pair variances on pair means), between- and within-pairs mean squares for each twin group are obtained by analysis of variance. Variance due to age-dependent regression is removed from the between-pairs mean squares and variance due to a mean difference between males and females removed from the opposite-sex within-pair mean square. Models may now be fitted to the corrected observed mean squares by the method of weighted least squares which produces approximately maximum likelihood parameter estimates and allows a χ^2 test of goodness-of-fit of the model.

Given the practical impossibility of detecting dominance in twin studies of most behavioral characters [Eaves, 1972; Martin et al, in press], the most usual models to be fitted are subsets of that shown in Table I. Here E_1 is the within-families environmental variation which includes environmental experiences specific to the individual and errors of measurement, and D_R is the additive genetic variance component defined by Mather and Jinks [1971]. The third parameter B is a between-families component of variance in which between-families environmental variation E_2 (cultural and family treatment effects) is completely confounded with the extra additive genetic variation which accrues between families as a result of assortative mating. This confounding can be seen in the expression:

$$B = E_2 + \frac{1}{2} D_R \left[\frac{A}{1-A} \right],$$

TABLE I. Basic Model for Mean Squares of a
Classical Twin Study

	E_1	B	D_R
MZF[a]			
b	1	2	1
w	1	0	0
MZM			
b	1	2	1
w	1	0	0
DZF			
b	1	2	¾
w	1	0	¼
DZM			
b	1	2	¾
w	1	0	¼
DZO			
b	1	2	¾
w	1	0	¼

[a]Abbreviations: MZF, monozygous female; MZM,
monozygous male; DZF, dizygous female, DZM,
dizygous male; DZO, dizygous opposite sexes;
b, between; w, within. Other abbreviations defined
in text.

where A is the correlation between the additive deviations of spouses and is related
to the phenotypic marital correlation μ by $A = h^2\mu$, where h^2 is the narrow
heritability.

When significant estimates of both D_R and B are obtained, we cannot even
guess at the relative contributions of E_2 and assortative mating to $\hat{B}$ without some
independent evidence about the size of marital correlation.

A more fundamental statistical question arises when we consider the power of
our experiment to reject inappropriate models of variation. There is no general
solution to this problem, so we must calculate the probability of rejecting inappropriate models of variation with samples of given size taken from imaginary
populations whose true components of variation are known. These calculations
are based upon the noncentral χ^2 distribution and are explained in detail in
Martin et al [in press]. We shall consider only a few of their results, shown here
in Table II. This table shows, for example, that in twin samples consisting of 50%
MZ and 50% DZ pairs drawn from a population in which the "true" components
of variation were one-half E_1 and one-half E_2, 430 pairs (215 MZ and 215 DZ)
would be required to reject an inappropriate $E_1 V_A$ ($V_A = 1/2D_R$) model at the
5% level of significance in 95% of such studies, while in the converse case, 640

TABLE II. Total Number of Pairs Required for 95% Rejection of False Hypotheses at 5% Level

True model			False model P (MZ)				
			0.1	0.3	0.5	0.7	0.9
$0.5E_1$	$0.5E_2$	E_1V_A	298	324	430	696	2,055
$0.5E_1$	$0.5V_A$	E_1E_2	2,181	852	640	670	1,344
		E_1E_2	1,798	660	466	455	848
$0.4V_A$	$0.3E_1$	$0.3E_2$					
		E_1V_A	645	718	966	1,583	4,715

pairs would be required to reject an inappropriate E_1E_2 model when the population variance is one-half E_1 and one-half additive genetic. In general it is easier to reject an inappropriate simple genetic (E_1V_A) model than an inappropriate simple environmental (E_1E_2) model in equivalent cases.

In the lower part of Table II we consider a more complex case in which the true population variance is attributable roughly one-third each to additive genetic, E_1, and between family (E_2 or assortative mating) sources. In this case we want to know the sample sizes required to reject (in 95% of studies at the 5% level) both the inappropriate two-parameter models. For all reasonable sample compositions it is easier to reject the E_1E_2 model than the E_1V_A model, although, with roughly one-third MZ pairs, 95% power of rejection of both models can be achieved with around 700 pairs. For 50% MZ twins, however, roughly twice as many twins are required to achieve 95% power of rejection of the E_1V_A model (966 pairs) as are needed to reject the E_1E_2 model (466 pairs). This is the approximate composition of the three twin samples we shall be considering. In this connection it is worth noting that, for these experiments, roughly 80% power can be achieved with samples around two-thirds the size of these and roughly 50% power with samples around one-third these sample sizes.

RESULTS AND DISCUSSION

With these power considerations in mind, we may now consider the results of model fitting to the data. The mean squares for Radicalism from the three twin studies (measured on three different scales) are shown in Table III, and the goodness-of-fit of various models fitted to these data is shown in Table IV.

It can be seen that the E_1E_2 model is decisively rejected in studies I and III and gives a very poor account of the data in study II (where the sample size is smallest). The simple genetic (E_1D_R) model is rejected in study I, fails marginally in

TABLE III. Observed Mean Squares From Three Twin Studies of Radicalism

	Study I (823 pairs)		Study II (246 pairs)		Study III (587 pairs)	
	DF	MS	DF	MS	DF	MS
MZF_b	323	8.36	93	337.97	231	112.92
w	324	1.90	95	61.50	233	24.95
MZM_b	141	10.31	37	356.52	81	113.77
w	142	1.78	39	49.20	83	30.02
DZF_b	193	9.51	52	365.26	145	121.84
w	194	2.89	54	100.83	147	39.17
DZM_b	36	8.85	15	272.48	50	124.96
w	37	3.21	17	82.38	52	44.89
DZO_b	126	10.11	39	350.61	70	128.16
w	126	3.29	41	129.35	72	49.11

TABLE IV. Results of Model Fitting for Radicalism

	Study I	Study II	Study III
E_1E_2 model $\chi^2_8 =$	24.74**	15.17*	21.03**
E_1D_R model $\chi^2_8 =$	20.61**	7.70	14.28*
E_1D_RB model $\chi^2_7 =$	7.51	3.26	6.20

*0.05 < P < 0.10.
**0.001 < P < 0.01.

study III, but gives an adequate account in study II. Clearly studies I and III indicate the need for all three parameters in an adequate model, and this gives an excellent fit to the data in the two largest studies. Although the third parameter is not strictly needed in study II, it does cause a significant reduction in the residual chi-square ($\chi^2_1 = 4.4$), justifying its inclusion in the model.

The congruence of these three studies is even more marked when we examine the breakdown of the total variation shown in Table V.

In each study, roughly one-third of the variation is attributable to within-family environmental variation (E_1), one-third to additive genetic (V_A), and one-third to a between-family component (B) which may be E_2 or additional genetic variation due to assortative mating, or both.

The only leverage we can get on this question is various estimates of the phenotypic marital correlation (μ) for the Radical-Conservative dimension obtained for

TABLE V. Sources of Variance for Radicalism (%)

	Study I	Study II	Study III
E_1	33.3	27.3	35.1
V_A	35.4	44.3	37.6
B $\Big\langle$ E_2	15.7	0.0	18.6
B	31.3	28.4	27.3
$\Big\rangle$ A.M.	15.6	28.4	8.7
	($\mu = 0.60$)	($\mu = 0.67$)	($\mu = 0.40$)

the three scales from independently collected husband-wife samples. These were $\hat{\mu} = 0.60$ for the scale used in study I, $\hat{\mu} = 0.67$ for the scale used in study II, and $\hat{\mu} = 0.40$ for the scale used in study III. It might be argued that these remarkably high correlations arise from a convergence of opinions over the years of marriage. We had no direct test of this but were able to regress absolute husband-wife differences on mean pair age (presumably a reasonable index of length of marriage) and, over quite a wide age range, found no significant regression. It appears, then, that the high marital correlation is a good reflection of the degree of assortative mating for this trait rather than of convergence of attitudes. If we substitute these values of $\hat{\mu}$ and the estimates of D_R into

$$A = h^2\mu$$
$$= \frac{\mu([1/2]D_R [1 + A/(1 - A)])}{\hat{V}_T} ,$$

where $\hat{V}_T = \hat{E}_1 + \hat{B} + (1/2) \hat{D}_R$, we can obtain estimates of A and hence $(1/2)D_R A/(1 - A)$ and (by subtraction from B) E_2. This breakdown has been done for each of three studies and is shown at the bottom of Table V. The figures show that all of B could be accounted for by assortative mating in study II (the least reliable), one-quarter in study III, and about one-half in study I. These figures would raise the heritability to around 50%, while "true" E_2 due to cultural influences and parental transmission would account for perhaps less than one-fifth of the total variation. However, to obtain stronger evidence on these points, data on the parents of twins and on adopted families will be needed. These data are currently being collected and analyzed in our laboratory.

For Radicalism, there is no evidence that genetic and environmental components of variation are not the same in males and females. When we inspect the mean squares for Toughmindedness shown in Table VI, however, it appears that,

TABLE VI. Sex Differences in Genetic Architecture

| | Toughmindedness | | | | Libido | |
| | Study I (823 pairs) | | Study II (246 pairs) | | | |
	DF	MS	DF	MS	DF	MS
MZF_b	323	10.37	93	383.2	93	312.9
w	324	1.86	95	79.5	93	125.2
MZM_b	141	7.82	37	391.0	37	376.0
w	142	3.20	39	93.4	39	93.0
DZF_b	193	7.52	52	248.9	52	272.4
w	194	3.00	54	125.1	54	99.8
DZM_b	36	6.57	15	548.8	15	312.4
w	37	3.37	17	62.9	17	155.4
DZO_b	126	8.13	39	299.1	39	287.3
w	126	4.32	41	148.6	41	180.8

while genetic components of variation are important in females, there is no such evidence in males. Inspection of the mean squares for the attitude trait Libido suggests exactly the reverse, with a strong cultural effect acting in females but a genetic component important in males. These traits both suggest some sort of sex limitation of cultural and genetic effects.

Eaves [1977] has provided a model for such sex-limited effects which is shown in complete form in Table VII. This model is not of full rank, and in any case, a parsimonious description would demand fewer parameters. There are many possible sensible subsets of these parameters, and there is a real danger of fitting them all and picking the one that fits best. Let us, however, formalize our observation that there appears to be no genetic variation for Toughmindedness in males, nor for Libido in females, but allow E_2 variation in both sexes. The results of fitting these models are shown in Table VIII.

The models give an excellent fit to the data in all three cases. For both studies of Toughmindedness there is a large and significant additive genetic component for females with a correspondingly small E_2 component, while for males the E_2 component is large. For both Toughmindedness and Libido in study II the total variances for males and females have been deliberately equalized. This has not been done in study I which explains why different E_1 components are needed for males and females.

The component $\hat{E}_{2MF}$ is an estimate of the covariance between E_2 effects acting in males and E_2 effects acting in females. Consequently $r_{MF} = E_{2MF}/(E_{2M}, E_{2F})^{\frac{1}{2}}$ is a measure of the correlation between E_2 effects acting in males and females. It can be seen from the model that this information comes from the opposite-sex pairs and emphasizes the importance of including these

results to sampling error, but they happen to be exactly the pattern of mean squares expected to be produced by the genetic effects of competition between siblings. If the extent to which sibs compete for a limited resource is dependent upon their genetic similarity, then it is evident that competition will be much more intense within MZ pairs than within DZ pairs. Consequently, variation between MZ pairs will tend to decrease relative to variation between DZ twins, and to the extent that the competition has a genetic basis, variance within DZ pairs will increase. These considerations are developed and formalized by Eaves [1976], who provides the model shown in Table IX, and fitted to the data for Sexual Satisfaction. The parameter $D_R{}'$ is almost significantly negative indicating the presence of a large competition effect based upon genetic similarity — a kind of genotype-environment covariation. This case is discussed more fully by Martin and Eysenck [1976] and Eaves [1977], but in verbal terms we may suggest that female twins are competing for male attention and that this competition is more intense among MZ females (where the male has a real dilemma) than among DZ females (where presumably the choice is usually more obvious). Since success in the competition has a genetic component, genetic differences will play a more important part among DZ females, and this explains the higher heritability for DZ twins than for MZ twins shown in Table IX.

The most important point to take from this case, however, is that there can be a rational genetic explanation for unequal MZ and DZ total variances and for negative intraclass correlations.

REFERENCES

Eaves LJ (1972): Computer simulation of sample size and experimental design in human psychogenetics. Psychol Bull 77:144−152.

Eaves LJ (1976): A model for sibling effects in man. Heredity 36:205−214.

Eaves LJ (1977): Inferring the causes of human variation. J Roy Statist Soc A, 140.

Eaves LJ, Eysenck HJ (1974): Genetics and the development of of social attitudes. Nature 249: 288−289.

Eaves LJ, Eysenck HJ (1975): The nature of extraversion: A genetical analysis. J Personal Soc Psychol 32:102−112.

Eaves LJ, Last KA, Martin NG, Hewitt JK, Eysenck HJ (in preparation): The causes of individual differences in social attitudes.

Eysenck HJ (1976): "Sex and Personality." London: Open Books.

Hewitt JK (1974): An analysis of data from a twin study of social attitudes. Unpublished MS Thesis, University of Birmingham, England.

Kasriel J, Eaves LJ (1976): A comparison of the accuracy of written questionnaires with blood-typing for diagnosing zygosity in twins. J Biosoc Sci 8:263−266

Last KA (in preparation): Unpublished PhD Thesis, University of Birmingham, England.

Martin NG (1975): The inheritance of scholastic abilities in a sample of twins. II. Genetic analysis of examination results. Ann Hum Genet 39:219−229.

Martin NG (1977): The classical twin study in human behaviour genetics. PhD Thesis, University of Birmingham, England.

Martin NG, Eysenck HJ (1976): Genetic factors in sexual behaviour. In Eysenck HJ:

"Sex and Personality." London: Open Books.

Martin NG, Eaves LJ, Eysenck HJ (1977): Genetical, environmental and personality factors influencing the age of first sexual intercourse in twins. J Biosoc Sci 9:91–97.

Martin NG, Eaves LJ, Kearsey MJ, Davies P (in press): The power of the classical twin study. Heredity.

Mather K, Jinks JL (1971): "Biometrical Genetics." 2nd Ed. London: Chapman and Hall.

Wilson G (1973): "The Psychology of Conservatism." London: Academic Press.

Temperaments in Twins

Steven G Vandenberg and Allan R Kuse

Most European languages have four adjectives descriptive of particular temperaments, inherited from medieval modification of Greek and Roman concepts about relationships between body fluids and constitution. These adjectives are the following:

Melancholic, a person with an excess of black bile, having a somewhat somber, slowly reacting disposition. In extreme cases this was thought to lead to what now is called depression. In Robert Burton's (1577–1640) "Anatomy of Melancholia" [1621] it is equated with all types of mental illness.

Sanguine, a person in whom blood predominates. Such persons react eagerly and energetically, tend to be even-tempered and optimistic.

Choleric, a person with an excess of choler (yellow bile), a substance no longer recognized in modern medicine. Such persons are quick to become angry or enthusiastic, and quickly forget again and lose interest.

Phlegmatic, a person who is slow to react, but persistent, even-tempered and giving the impression of being somewhat cold.

We will use in this paper the conceptions of temperaments or basic personality constellations of a Dutch psychologist, Gerard J. Heymans (1857–1930).

Heymans thought that these four adjectives were useful and that their generality in western Europe suggested that they had some valid basis, perhaps biological in origin. He took these four typologic concepts and after adding four new types came up with a reinterpretation, converting the typology to a system with three quantitative bipolar traits. He dropped the melancholic type, possibly because of its connotations of abnormality. In his modernizing effort he seems to have

Twin Research: Psychology and Methodology, pages 25–31
© **1978 Alan R. Liss, Inc., New York, N.Y.**

attempted to line up these dimensions with three basic functions: cognition, emotion, and volition or conation. Heymans redefined the functions slightly so that they became maximally compatible with the endpoints of a three-dimensional personality cube represented by the eight adjectives. This cube is shown in Figure 1. The four additional types added by Heymans he called passionate, emotional, nervous, and amorphous. The three bipolar dimensions which Heymans envisioned are discussed next.

The dimension representing cognition is not identical with intelligence as we think of it today; after all, these ideas were worked out before Binet's scale was published. The term chosen by Heymans was secondary function, a concept borrowed from Otto Gross [1902], who used this expression to characterize the evolutionary trend towards increased freedom of choice, as various species with more complex nervous systems are behaving less and less under the control of built-in, fixed tropisms, reflexes, reponse tendencies, or "instincts." In primates and particularly in man, long delays in response are possible which, while preventing an immediate reaction, permit past experiences to influence responses to current events (see Stenhouse [1974] for a general discussion of the evolution of this aspect of intelligence and Elliot [1969] for the underlying evolution of the nervous system). The opposite of secondary function is primary function. (The reader will note the similarity to Freud's concepts of primary reactions controlled by the id and the pleasure-pain principle, and secondary reactions in which gratification is delayed because ego and especially superego functions intervene. A somewhat similar distinction is made by Russian physiologists and psychologists when they distinguish

HEYMANS' PERSONALITY TYPES

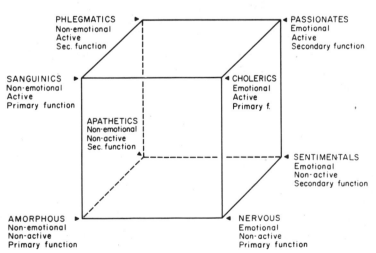

Fig. 1. A diagram of Heymans' three-dimensional personality theory, with the eight types listed at the corners.

between the primary and secondary signaling systems. According to Pavlov, the latter is associated in man with language and reflexion.)

According to Heymans (and Gross) persons high in secondary function display more long-range planning, stick with particular interests longer, and are less influenced by momentary fluctuations in their environment. Studies in which judges rate the personality of others often come up with a factor called dependability [Vernon, 1964]. It is likely that this is the same or a highly similar dimension.

The second dimension is emotionality, which runs from high to low. Heymans used this term not so much to describe volatile, moody, unstable, or neurotic behavior but partly referred to the controlled, even display of social attachment, the depth of feeling or commitment, and the warmth of affection. Nevertheless, some of the individual questions deal with the earlier-mentioned characteristics. The choice of this term may today seem somewhat awkward but in Heymans's system a highly (or strongly) emotional person would be one who forms strong attachments to particular persons, causes, and ideas and who is not ashamed to show it. There is therefore little suggestion of abnormality except perhaps in certain combinations with other traits. As a matter of fact, Heymans initially gave very little thought to implications of his ideas for psychiatry, although he later collaborated with the psychiatrist Wiersma. This dimension is therefore distinctly different from "nervousness" as in Eysenck's personality questionnaire, or in current popular usage. However, Heymans used the term "nervous" for one of his eight extremes, to typify a person low in activity and low in follow-through (primary rather than secondary function) but high in emotionality. The dimension is different also from Jung's concept of introversion-extraversion because one can be shallow and cold inside or have quickly changing interests or attractions but yet be classified as extravert without falling at the high end of the emotionality scale.

The third dimension is called active-nonactive. By activity Heymans meant vital energy — purposeful, sustained activity or perhaps biologic vigor rather than the restlessness one sometimes sees in individuals who are bored, tense, or upset. Nor should it be mistaken for the obsessive-compulsive need to keep busy, as for instance with constant housecleaning, doing calculations over and over, or working on one's car to keep it perfect and spotless. The other end of this dimension is characterized by easy fatigability, lack of energy, and so on. Of course the quality of the work produced as the result of the activity is partly determined by the intelligence of the person, but this is conceptually unrelated to the dimensions Heymans had in mind. Leaving aside the question to what extent these three dimensions are empirically independent, we will now return to the eight "typologic" extremes.

Using the three bipolar dimensions Heymans fitted the eight adjectives mentioned above to the following combinations of highs and lows. The eight extremes were raised by Heymans to the dimensions in the manner shown in Table I.

TABLE I. Heymans's Labels for the Nine Types Representing the Combinations of Extremes on the Three Bipolar Dimensions

Emotionality	Activity	Primary vs secondary function	Type
High	High	Secondary	Passionates
High	High	Primary	Cholerics
High	Low	Secondary	Sentimentals
High	Low	Primary	Nervous
Low	High	Secondary	Phlegmatics
Low	High	Primary	Sanguinics
Low	Low	Secondary	Apathetics
Low	Low	Primary	Amorphous

Before 1906 Heymans developed a questionnaire, a detailed description of which was not published until 1948, which he designated to measure these three dimensions after he had read and annotated a number of biographies of famous persons, noting mention of various behaviors and attributes of these individuals, and looking for co-occurrence of such items. This questionnaire was administered in two large studies, the results of which were published in Dutch, French, but mostly in German psychological journals before and during World War I (1906–1918). As the result of this timing, these papers received less attention than they might otherwise have received. In addition, the Zeitgeist was not quite ready for an interest in this type of "quantitative" approach. Nevertheless, Heymans's psychological work was noted by Cattell, Eysenck, and a few other persons and influenced some French psychologists such as LeSenne [1946], Maistriaux [1959], and Berger [1950, 1962].

In another paper we will summarize a French, a Belgian, and a Dutch study of Heymans's typology. In this one we will report preliminary results of a study of 79 pairs of MZ twins and 85 pairs of DZ twins.

The twins were recruited through the public school system in Louisville, Kentucky, and were all in high school. They were aged 12 through 18. There were 39 female and 40 male MZ pairs, and 23 female, 15 male, and 47 opposite-sex DZ pairs. Standardized factor scores for a three-factor solution were calculated using factor coefficients derived from a sample of 200 undergraduate college students. A three-factor solution is suggested by Heymans's theory. In a later paper we will discuss whether the data support this view of three independent factors or whether more factors seem to be represented in the responses to the questionnaire. For the purposes of this report we will accept the three-dimensional solution as an adequate condensation of the responses.

Table II summarizes the within-pair and between-pair variances for the five kinds of twins, while Table III shows the estimates of heritability obtained using

TABLE II. Within-Pair and Between-Pair Variances for Five Kinds of Twin Pairs

	Variance		
	Within pair	Between pair	Intraclass correlation
Monozygous males			
Factor I	0.440	0.911	0.35
Factor II	0.438	0.417	−0.03
Factor III	0.203	0.608	0.50
Monozygous females			
Factor I	0.235	0.803	0.55
Factor II	0.487	0.784	0.23
Factor III	0.263	0.547	0.35
All monozygous			
Factor I	0.339	0.847	0.43
Factor II	0.463	0.594	0.12
Factor III	0.233	0.646	0.47
Dizygous males			
Factor I	0.405	0.406	0.00
Factor II	0.307	0.559	0.29
Factor III	0.113	0.408	0.57
Dizygous females			
Factor I	0.466	0.805	0.27
Factor II	0.637	0.560	−0.07
Factor III	0.325	0.255	−0.12
All dizygous			
Factor I	0.396	0.662	0.25
Factor II	0.406	0.620	0.21
Factor III	0.289	0.433	0.20
Opposite sex pairs			
Factor I	0.359	0.657	0.29
Factor II	0.324	0.687	0.36
Factor III	0.327	0.527	0.23

Falconer's formula $2(r_{MZ} - r_{DZ})$. When a negative value was obtained it is indicated by an asterisk.

There is consistent and rather strong indication of a genetic component in the first factor which is characterized by the following type of statements:

I don't like to commit myself quickly on an issue.
I am not good at telling jokes.
It takes me a long time to get over a loss.
I am not good at finding a quick solution in a new and different situation.

This is clearly the secondary function described by Heymans. It may be noted that one of the questions deals with the lasting effect of a loss, which might be taken as an indication of emotionality. However, the next factor seems to be one clearly

TABLE III. Estimates of Heritability for Three Temperamental Factors Assessed by Heymans's Questionnaire

Factor I (Secondary function)	
Males	0.70
Females	0.56
Total	0.36
Factor II (Emotionality)	
Males	*
Females	0.46
Total	*
Factor III (Activity)	
Males	*
Females	0.70
Total	0.54

*Negative values obtained.

representing at least some aspects of emotionality, although the items having the highest factor loadings refer more to undesirable aspects (referred to above as "nervousness") than to the strong commitment which characterized Heymans's conception. Examples of high-loading questions are:

I am easily upset.
I am not handy with tools.
I lose my temper easily.

There is no consistent evidence from this study of a genetic component in this factor because the intraclass correlation was 0.29 for the dizygous males and −0.03 for the monozygous males, although the situation was reversed for the females: 0.23 for the MZ and −0.07 for the DZ, which suggests a genetic factor for the females but not the males. This could in part be due to a different reaction by females than by males either to questions or to the life situations which the questions attempt to sample. However, there are no significant sex differences to any of the items and the interclass correlations of the opposite-sex twins for this factor is 0.36, which is higher than the value for the other two dimensions.

For the third factor the same result was found, ie, no evidence of a genetic component in males but only in females. Here, however, it is not a matter of a lack of similarity of the MZ males (r 0.50), but rather an equally high similarity for the DZ males (r 0.57), while for females these values were 0.35 and −0.12. This third factor is characterized by items such as the response:

"I like to keep busy" and by affirmative answers to questions having to do with active hobbies. Apparently this is Heymans's activity factor.

When the data for males and females are combined, there is a suggestion of a genetic component for the activity dimension. Further analyses are planned in which the twin resemblance will be considered for other subsets of questions which may define additional factors but not proposed by Heymans.

This is not the place for an extended discussion of the factor analysis in which we employed three factors. Suffice it to say here that the replication of Heymans's factors was not as clear-cut as we would have liked. This may in part contribute to the inconclusive evidence about genetic contributions to the three factors.

SUMMARY

Responses of identical and fraternal twins to a personality questionnaire developed by Heymans were compared for evidence of a genetic component in the three major personality factors proposed by Heymans. There was substantial evidence of a genetic component for both males and females in factor I which represents secondary function. For factor II, emotionality, only the results for the females, but not for the males, were compatible with a genetic component. The same results were obtained for factor III, activity. Further analyses are planned.

REFERENCES

Berger G (1950): "Traité practique d'analyse du caractère." Paris: Presses Universitaires de France.

Berger G (1962): Caractère et personnalité. Paris: Presses Universitaires de France.

Burton R (1621): "Anatomy of Melancholia." New York: Random House (1932 edition by JM Dent, London, reissued 1977.)

Elliot HC (1969): "The Shape of Intelligence: The Evolution of the Human Brain." New York: Scribner's.

Bross O (1902): "Die cerebrale Sekundarfunktion." Vogel: Leipzig.

Heymans GJ (1906—1918): Beiträge zur speciellen Psychologie auf Grund einer Massenuntersuchung [Contribution to differential psychology based on a massive survey]. Psychol 42, pp 81—127, 258—301; 43, pp 321—373; 45, pp 1—42; 46, pp 321—333; 51, 1—72; 62, pp 1—59; 80, pp 76—89.

Heymans GJ (1908): Uber einige psychischen Korrelationen [on some psychological correlations]. Z Angew Psychol 1:313—381.

Heymans GJ (1948): "Inleiding tot de speciale psychologie" [Introduction to differential psychology]. Haarlem, Netherlands: Bohn.

LeSenne R (1946): "Traité de caractérologie." Paris: Presses Universitaires de France.

Maistriaux R (1959): "Intelligence et la caractère." Paris: Presses Universitaires de France.

Stenhouse D (1974): "The Evolution of Intelligence." London: Allen & Unwin.

Vernon PE (1964): "Personality Assessment, A Critical Survey." London: Methuen.

Revelations of the Electra Complex and Sibling Rivalry in the Kinetic Family Drawings of Seven-Year-Old Identical Twin Girls

Josef E Garai and Jo Anne Frohock

INTRODUCTION

In the present work, the Kinetic Family Drawing Test was used with one set of 7-year-old identical twin girls. The results indicate that twinship appears to pose problems far more intense than with other sib relationships in the areas of personal identity, sib rivalry, and the development of sexual identity through the challenge of the transitional Electra stage. Similar test results with other identical twin girls of this age have been obtained [Garai, unpublished]. Based on these findings, it is possible to conclude that there is a strong similarity between identical twins in primary-process thinking

The Kinetic Family Drawing (K-F-D) Test was developed by Burns and Kaufman [1970, 1972]. It is a nonverbal diagnostic technique for uncovering disturbances related to family interactions. Garai [unpublished] modifies the test as follows: 1) The client is supplied with at least 12 different colored crayons instead of a pencil. Past research by Hammer [1969] indicates that the forced use of color elicits more spontaneous and fewer defensive responses; 2) Burns and Kaufman's instructions to the client, "Draw a picture of everyone in your family, including you, doing something," is replaced here by the instruction "Draw a picture of *a* family doing something." The latter instruction reduces anxiety and allows for revealing omissions or modifications of family members in the projection as it compares with the actual family of the client. Other interpretations are based

Twin Research: Psychology and Methodology, pages 33—41

on techniques developed by Buck and Hammer [1966]; Buck and Hammer [1969]; Hammer [1969]; Garai [unpublished], and Machover [1949]. The protocol used at the end of the test is as follows:

1. Give the age, sex and family status of each member of this family.

2. What is each one doing?

3. How does each member like what he/she is doing?

4. What else would each member like to be doing?

5. Who is the happiest member in the family?

6. Who is the unhappiest member of the family?

7. Make up a story about this family.

AN ILLUSTRATIVE CASE

Geraldine and Nina are 7-year-old identical twin girls who have lived all their lives in New York City. Their 46-year-old father works as a waiter in a French restaurant, having come to this country from France as an adult. He is dissatisfied with his work, has few friends, and claims 95% of his emotional investment is in his wife and the twins — though work keeps him away from them much of the time. The mother in the family is 40 years old, American-born, and Jewish. She and the father both claim she is the most dominant member of the family. Neither feels happy with their sex life. She claims she does not "feel sexual" often enough. He feels inadequate in his efforts to please her. The twins spend most of their time with their mother, as their father works nights and has to sleep much of the day. The parents have different feelings about the twins. The mother claims to admire Geraldine most, as Geraldine is independent and has more highly developed verbal skills. (The mother wishes she had become a writer herself.) The mother claims however, that she never really felt she gave birth to Geraldine, who was the later born of the seven-weeks-premature twins and was not expected to live during the first three days of life. The mother identifies with Nina's sensitivity and dependence. The father simply claims to feel closer to whichever twin needs him most at a given time. The parents dress the twins differently and have them in different classes at school in order to help the girls develop as individuals. The parents would like the twins to be bilingual, so the father speaks to them only in French. The twins understand well enough, but they always answer him in English. The mother claims to have studied Spanish, but she speaks only English. She says that as infants the twins probably did not get enough "holding." Consequently, Geraldine still sleeps with a security blanket and Nina with two pacifiers.

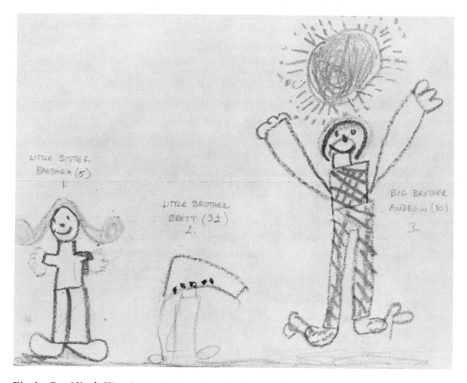

LITTLE SISTER
BARBARA (5)
1.

LITTLE BROTHER
BRETT (3½)
2.

BIG BROTHER
ANDREW (10)
3.

Fig. 1. Geraldine's Kinetic Family Drawing (family members numbered in the order they were drawn): 1) little sister, Barbara, aged 5 years; 2. little brother, Brett, aged 3½ years; and 3) big brother, Andrew, aged 10 years.

Geraldine's K-F-D

There is an unusual amount of obsessive-compulsive behavior exhibited by Geraldine in the completion of her drawing. She delays 20 seconds before even beginning her drawing, asks if she can have a pencil with an eraser rather than crayons, and seems baffled and dissatisfied with her efforts to draw and unable to think up ideas. Repeatedly the investigator has to encourage her not to worry about mistakes and to draw anything she wishes. Not until the end of the protocol when she is asked to tell a story about the family does she seem confident.

Geraldine does not deal with any of the members of her family in a direct way. This includes herself. Instead of a mother, father, and two twin sisters, she draws a sister younger than herself by two years, a much younger brother, and an older brother. The little sister is the one she most identifies as herself. She projects feelings about Nina, her twin sister, onto Brett, the 3½-year-old little brother in

TABLE I. Protocol (Geraldine)

I. Age, sex, family status of each member of this family
   1. Little sister (Barbara) — 5 years
   2. Little brother (Brett) — 3½ years
   3. Big brother (Andrew) — 10 years

II. What is each one doing?
   1. Laughing at both of the others.
   2. Looking for something with his head in his jacket.
   3. Trying to reach the sun, though it might burn his hands.

III. How does each member like what he/she is doing?
   1. Barbara likes to laugh at them a lot.
   2. Brett doesn't like what he is doing because his head was stuck in his jacket
      and he was trying to get it out, and he was looking for something. (Laughs)
      He doesn't like it at all!
   3. Andrew will feel disappointed if he doesn't reach the sun because he wanted to
      to be the first one to reach it. (Laughs) To be the first one to burn his hands!

IV. What else would each member like to be doing?
   1. Painting a picture.
   2. Swinging on the swings in the park.
   3. In the park playing freeze-tag.

V. Who is the happiest member of the family?
   Barbara

VI. Who is the unhappiest member of the family?
   Brett

VII. Make up a story about this family.
   (See text.)

the picture. The 10-year-old brother, Andrew, is clearly the way she deals with her father. There are ambivalence and evasiveness here. She is reluctant to draw anyone after she draws Barbara, which indicates self-concern or egocentrism. Yet Barbara is seen as passive, dependent, and insecure. Geraldine says, "There is nothing Barbara can do because her hands are not long enough to reach the sun." So Barbara just stands there and laughs at the others. Barbara's short arms point to a feeling of helplessness; the yellow color of the hands indicates hostility. A feeling of overdependency is shown in Barbara's long neck. Insecurity is manifested in the heavy ground line and oversized feet of Barbara. Most interesting in Geraldine's drawing is the omission of a mother figure. The huge, hot sun is probably a symbolic representation of her mother. It is what her self-identified figure would like to reach but cannot; it is what her father-identified figure may be the first to reach — but only to get his hands burned while she, Geraldine, scorns and resents him (note the way she "X-es out" Andrew's body). The story she tells about the family she draws is as follows:

> All stories start 'Once upon a time,' so this will start 'One day,' I guess.
> One day Andrew went fishing. And Barbara keeps telling Brett to push him
> into the water, but Brett did not know what that meant. So Barbara told
> him and he said: 'No!' Then Barbara said that it would be funny because he
> wouldn't catch any fish and he would get all wet. So Brett pushed him into
> the water and he was really angry at him. So he hit him on the head with a
> hammer. Then Brett started to cry. Then Barbara told Brett to stop crying
> because it was a sponge hammer but Brett cried anyway. Then Andrew
> started teasing both of them and they started pushing him. And Andrew
> started running after them and they went far, far away, and they never
> stopped. But one day they did stop. And that time when they stopped,
> Andrew was 146 years old. And Geraldine was 40, I guess. No, Barbara
> was 40. And Brett was about 7 years old – no, 21. And then they never
> ran again. You know why? 'Cause they couldn't. They were dead because
> an old man with a big, long, heavy sword cut their heads off, and they
> tried to run away, but they couldn't. And that was the end of all of them.

Nina's K-F-D

Nina executes her Kinetic Family Drawing in 5 minutes, 40 seconds, showing less obsessive-compulsive defensiveness than Geraldine. She states that the
woman on the left with the red dress and blue belt is the mother, aged 25 and at
once corrects the age to 34. Next comes the baby brother, aged 4½, then the
big sister, aged 13, and the father, aged 39. They are having a picnic with picnic
baskets. Everyone is holding two things: the mother two sandwiches, the baby
brother two sandwiches, the sister a sandwich and an apple, and the father apple
juice and orange juice. Nina says the mother likes the country the most. The
other three would rather be in the city. The baby brother likes to fool around
with sticks and pull up grass. The sister likes to take big giant sticks and hit them
on the trees and try to break them. She also likes to find caterpillars a lot and
play with them. (Nina volunteers that she likes to do both herself.) The father
likes to just lie down in the grass and take a nap. Nina, when asked for a story
about the family, responds as follows:

> I don't know what to start with . . . (long pause). That's the most hardest
> part, thinking what to start with (long pause). I can't think of anything (long
> pause). Did Gerry have trouble thinking of something also or not? (pause).
> (After encouragement by the examiner to make up any story she wants,
> she continues.) Maybe I'll start with 'Once there was a family going on a
> trip to a picnic at Rye Beach. And the mother loved it; and the sister liked
> it second of all; and the father liked it third of all; and the baby brother
> liked it fourth of all. And after they ate lunch, they went down to the beach.
> And then later when they came home they ate dinner. They watched tele-
> vision a little bit and they went to bed.' They didn't do much that day,
> did they? But they stayed on the picnic a long time.

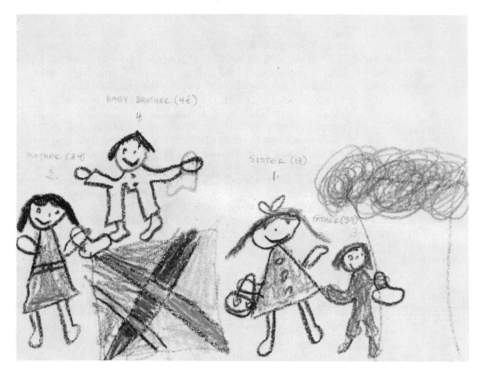

Fig. 2. Nina's Kinetic Family Drawing (family members numbered in the order they were drawn): 1) sister, aged 13 years; 2) mother, aged 34 years; 3) father, aged 39 years; and 4) baby brother, aged 4½ years.

Comparison of Drawings

Both twins see their mother as the most powerful member of the family, but they see their father as their chief source of nurturance. Each vies with the other for his affection, and each wishes to have him to herself and to get his attention turned away from the mother. Each would also like to punish him when he does not conform to this wish. Geraldine would also bring misfortune on the head of her twin, as well as transform her into a less threatening rival. She changes her identical twin sister into a younger brother. She excludes the mother figure from her picture altogether. Even so, the strong maternal presence creeps in, symbolized by the sun — a sun she herself cannot reach — a sun that will burn the hands of her father, symbolized by Andrew. Ambivalence over such yearnings is keen, as can be seen in the "beheading" of young Brett in the pic-

TABLE II. Protocol (Nina)

I. Age, sex, family status of each member of this family

    1. Big sister – 13 years
    2. Mother – 25, I mean 34 years
    3. Father – about 39 years
    4. Baby brother – 4½ years

II. What is each one doing?

    All are having a picnic and holding two things

    1. Sandwich and an apple
    2. Two sandwiches
    3. Apple juice and orange juice
    4. Two sandwiches

III. How does each member like what he/she is doing?

    1. The sister likes to take big giant sticks and hit them on the trees and tries to break them. (Laughs) That's what I would like to do.
    2. The mother likes the country a lot. She likes to go outside and have a picnic.
    3. He likes what he is doing right now.
    4. The baby brother likes to fool around with sticks and pull up grass. This is pretty fun to him.

IV. What else would each member like to be doing?

    1. Find caterpillars a lot and play with them. That's what I do there.
    2. She would rather be picnicking in Rye. My mother likes to go the the beach there.
    3. The father just likes to lay down in the grass and take a nap. That's what my daddy does.
    4. Ride his tricycle.

V. Who is the happiest member of the family?

    The mother, because she likes to picnic the best. And also, the other three people like it better in the city.

VI. Who is the unhappiest member of the family?

    The father, because he doesn't like to go picnicking very much.

VII. Make up a story about this family.
    (See text.)

---

ture and of all three in her story. Castration anxiety is strongly manifested in this symbolism. Nina simply places her "security" picnic blanket between her self-identified figure and the mother. She puts herself nearest the father and her sib nearest the mother – forming a mother/twin alliance and a father/twin alliance. Again, the twin sister becomes a younger brother.

The twins each seek to realize their Electra fantasies by the further magical alteration of ages in order to make the incestuous relationship more feasible. Geraldine makes her father into an older brother (Andrew), thereby removing the generation difference. Nina, on the other hand, transforms herself into an early 13-year-old adolescent girl. Then she rejuvenates her 46-year-old father into a 39-year-old man who is hanging onto her skirt. She has become the fully developed woman who replaces her mother. The primary process strategy of magical age and gender transformation is obviously used by both twins to reach the same end.

Geraldine and Nina each show a marked interest in things over people. Geraldine, in listing her own family members, gives the dog and cat equal status with the rest of the family. She further says she likes her mother best, because her mother buys her more *things*. Nina spends the major portion of her drawing time on the picnic blanket with its huge "X" of hot and cold colors, separating mother and daughter. This and then the tree are completed before the inclusion of any people in her picture.

Both girls are unusually expressive. However, each experiences extreme difficulty in the mode of expression that is the forte of the other. In other words, drawing the picture is almost impossible for Geraldine. Not until she begins her story, does she feel competent and eager. The very opposite is true with Nina. For her, the drawing is easy with the story coming painfully hard and only with the prodding of the examiner.

CONCLUSION

The fact that both twins seek to resolve their Electra complexes and feelings of competition with both an identical sib and an overstrong mother figure is not surprising. That they each employ almost identical strategies — namely, the magic of age and gender transformation — is striking. When the K-F-D was given to another set of 7-year-old identical twin girls each of the second pair chose the same strategies as the first, which is even more interesting. Certainly a larger sample needs to be run; but based on these preliminary findings, it would seem that being an identical twin intensifies some of the challenges of the developmental stages, as well as presenting problems unique to twins. Perhaps the phenomenon of identical twinship may probe to the very depths of primary-process thinking. This state of affairs may be so emotionally charged that it cannot reach into consciousness.

At any rate, the Kinetic Family Drawing Test seems to be an ideal instrument for revealing some of the hidden feelings twins have about themselves, their twins, and their relationships with the rest of their family.

REFERENCES

Buck JN (1966): "The House-Tree-Person Technique: Revised Manual." Beverly Hills, California: Western Psychological Services.

Buck JN, Hammer EF (eds) (1960): "Advances in the House-Tree-Personal Technique: Variations and Applications." Los Angeles: Western Psychological Services.

Burns RC, Kaufman SH (1970): "Kinetic Family Drawings (K-F-D): An Introduction to Understanding Children Through Kinetic Drawings." New York: Brunner/Mazel.

Burns RC, Kaufman SH (1972): "Actions, Styles and Symbols in Kinetic Family Drawings (K-F-D): An Interpretative Manual." New York: Brunner/Mazel.

Garai JE (Unpublished papers): Pratt Institute, Brooklyn, New York.

Hammer EF (1969): Hierarchal organization of personality and the H-T-P achromatic and chromatic. In Buck JN, Hammer EF (eds): "Advances in the House-Tree-Person Technique: Variations and Applications." Los Angeles: Western Psychological Serivces, chap 1, pp 1–35.

Machover K (1949): "Personality Projection in the Drawing of the Human Figure: A Method of Personality Investigation." Springfield, IL: Charles C Thomas.

Genetic Analysis of Twins' Naturalistically Observed Behavior

Hugh Lytton

The research on which this paper is based had as its main focus the effects of parents' child-rearing practices, as well as of genetic factors, on the development of compliance, attachment, independence, and speech. Naturalistic observations in the home (two three-hour sessions, one week apart) yielded detailed records in code of the interactions of 2.5-year-old male twins with their parents, from which behavior counts were derived. These were supplemented by interviews and ratings, as well as by experimental procedures in a playroom. The present paper reports the genetic analysis of the child's behavioral measures, and provides evidence on the differential treatment by parents of monozygotic (MZ) and dizygotic (DZ) twins.

The sample consisted of 17 MZ and 29 DZ male twin pairs — almost the total population of male sets of twins born in Calgary, Canada, during two successive years. As a control group, 44 male singletons were also included in the sample. The zygosity of the twins was ascertained by blood-typing *after* the psychological investigation was complete.

The behavior counts were summed for each child and expressed as rates per minute (eg, for speech) or as percentages of the child's total actions. Ratings were based on total impression during the observations, as well as on interview with the mother, and the playroom variables were scores assigned immediately after short experimental procedures. The Peabody Picture Vocabulary Test (PPVT) was administered during the experimental session. The interobserver reliability of behavior counts was only marginally satisfactory; the reliability of ratings and, particularly, of the experimental measures was, however, much higher. The method is described in detail in Lytton [1973].

Twin Research: Psychology and Methodology, pages 43—48

The 28 child variables that have been used in the major analyses of this project were subjected to a biometrical genetic analysis by N Martin and LJ Eaves of the University of Birmingham, England [Lytton et al., in press]. The assumptions and methods for this type of analysis are discussed in Jinks and Fulker [1970].

A basic assumption for the genetic analysis is equality of total variances between the MZ and DZ groups. Variables for which total variances were not equal were excluded from the analysis. Certain differences in means of variables between the two groups were due to differences in the mothers' education and, once this was taken into account, the only significant difference in means between MZ and DZ groups that remained was in "number of formboard pieces placed" (an experimental task). Where skewed distribution and kurtosis suggested the presence of G $\times$ E (genetic $\times$ environmental) interaction, a square-root transformation was carried out to remove the distortions of scale. However, this transformation made little difference to the results and the analysis on the untransformed data is therefore reported.

Table I shows the results of fitting different models to the data by the method of least squares. A plus sign indicates that the model fits; ie, the χ^2 for testing the observed mean squares against the mean squares expected under the model is *not* significant. The simplest model, E_1, tests the hypothesis that all the variance is a result of within-family environmental experiences, or error. This model fits only the data for four out of five experimental variables and for the Peabody Vocabulary Test. It is just these measures which must be in doubt: The experimental variables seem to have poor construct validity [Lytton, 1974], and the standardization of the PPVT for this age was problematic.

The other models shown test whether the addition of a between-family environmental component (E_2) or of an additive genetic component (D_R), or both, provides a better fit for the observed data. The $E_1 D_R$ model fails in a number of cases and generally gives a worse fit than the $E_1 E_2$ model. The latter fits every one of the variables. The $E_1 E_2 D_R$ model also fits every variable and in each case fits better than the $E_1 E_2$ model, as is to be expected since we are making use of more information to explain the variance. However, only for the instrumental independence rating and rate of speech does the $E_1 E_2 D_R$ fit the data so much better that the genetic component (D_R) shows up as significant. For many variables D_R is even slightly negative. Where the genetic component is positive, a biometric heritability estimate is given in Table I, and its significance level accords with that of D_R. The last column in Table I displays heritability estimates calculated by the Haseman and Elston [1970] formula. A comparison between the two heritability estimates, arrived at via different approaches, is instructive. The figures do, in fact, accord very closely. Both methods demonstrate a significant heritability for the same two variables. Where the heritability estimated by one method assumes an "impossible" value, it usually does the same under the other method, or else the heritability shown is near zero. In

TABLE I. Model Fitting and "Heritabilities" for Child Variables

Variable name		Model fits				"Heritabilities"	
		E_1[a]	E_1E_2	E_1D_R	$E_1E_2D_R$	Biometric $\frac{1}{2}D_R/(\frac{1}{2}D_R + E_1 + E_2)$	Haseman and Elston [1970] $2(MS_{WDZ} - MS_{WMZ})/\sigma^2_{Tot}$
IQ-PPVT		+	+	+	+	—	0.21
Comply ratio	C	—	+	+	+	0.32 ± 0.38	0.26
Positive action	CR	—	+	—	+	—	—
Negative action	CR	—	+	+	+	—	—
Attachment	CR	—	+	—	+	—	—
Speech	CR	—	+	+	+	$0.37* \pm 0.21$	0.39*
Command	CP	—	+	+	+	0.11 ± 0.24	0.10
Total activity	COM	—	+	—	+	—	—
Compliance	HR	—	+	+	+	0.07 ± 0.28	0.07
Attachment	HR	—	+	+	+	—	—
Independence	HR	—	+	+	+	$0.59** \pm 0.23$	0.58**
Speech maturity	HR	—	+	—	+	0.00	0.00
Internalized standards	HR	—	+	+	+	0.17 ± 0.29	0.15
Compliance	PR	+	+	+	+	0.02 ± 0.60	—
Attachment	PR	+	+	+	+	—	0.02
Independence	PR	+	+	+	+	—	—
Total activity	PR	+	+	+	+	0.90 ± 0.56	0.75
Number of form-board pieces	PR	—	+	+	+	—	—

[a]Abbreviations: C, count variable; CR, rate per minute; CP, % of child's actions; HR, home rating; PR, playroom variable; COM, composite standardized score; E_1, within-family environmental component; E_2, between-family environmental component; D_R, additive genetic component. A minus sign in "Heritabilities" columns indicates a negative heritability.
*p < 0.05.
**p < 0.01.

view of the lack of a widely accepted paradigm for the estimation of genetic contribution to the variance, such concordance is comfort, indeed. It should be noted that the assumption of equality of total variances between the MZ and DZ groups underlies both of these methods and this assumption was, in fact, met for the variables analyzed.

The genetic harvest from these measures of child behavior, however, is but meager: Only the independence rating and the speech rate (a count variable) show a significant genetic component. The latter variable has been shown to be sensitive to the effects of twinship as such, and to the effects of the mother's education. It is probably a more reliable predictor of later intelligence than the PPVT score, which is obtained in a test situation and is subject to considerable fluctuations for 2.5-year-old children.

The modest reliability between observers may partly explain the small proportion of genetic variation in the count variables, but the greater reliability of ratings and experimental measures did not produce greater genetic determination. Though the sample size was large for an ethological study, it was small for a genetic one, and this fact is likely to be another reason for the seeming unimportance of genetic factors in the variables under study.

For most of these child characteristics the largest portion of the variance was explained by differences between families. In small measure these differences were attributable to interobserver differences, but mainly they reflected varying child-rearing situations and differences in cultural milieu. The systematic differences between twins and singletons, for instance [Lytton et al., 1977], seem to be an expression of such environmental variations.

That parents treat MZ twin partners no more alike than they do DZ twins is a basic assumption of the twin method. The measures of parental behavior towards their twins, derived from direct observation, that were available in this study provided an opportunity to examine the question of possible differential treatment. The first step was to compare the within-pair variances of parent behavioral measures for MZ twins with those for DZ twins. In 7 out of 48 such measures, the MZ variance was in fact significantly smaller; ie, parents treated MZ twins more alike than they did DZ twins. This occurred, for instance, for the mothers' use of material rewards, support of dependence, and encouragement of independence.

However, this greater similarity may not be a result of a stereotype of MZ twins having to be treated alike, but may be a reaction to the greater genetic similarity of MZ twins. I therefore separated out those parent actions which were not directly elicited by a child action — called "parent-initiated actions." If in such parent-initated actions, which are freed of the influence of the child's immediate behavior, parents do *not* treat MZ twins more alike, it can be argued that this suggests that parent behavior is not in general influenced by a stereotype of MZ likeness. The within-pair variances of parent-initiated actions for MZ twins were therefore compared with those for DZ twins (Table II). Action categories such as "suggestion" (eg, "Would you like to . . .?") or generally "positive action" were used for this purpose. Only for the mothers' use of suggestion was the DZ variance significantly larger than the MZ variance; for the other categories the DZ variances were either only slightly larger or actually smaller. In view of such random fluctuations in the within-pair variances, it would appear that parents do not, of their own accord and systematically, institute more similar treatment for MZ than for DZ twins.

Some more subjective evidence on the question comes from the interviews with the mothers. They were asked whether they made any deliberate differences between the twins and, if so, why they did so. Many mothers of both MZ and DZ twins acknowledge that they treated each twin differently, but they always attributed such differential treatment to the differing needs of the children, eg, saying that one child needed more warmth or was more mischievous, etc. (Such remarks may, of course, be rationalizations.)

The last procedure employed in investigating this question was based on Scarr's [1968] work. Like Scarr, I compared mothers' attitudes toward, and treatment of, twin pairs about whose zygosity the mother was mistaken. Four pairs in my sample were thought by the mother to be DZ, when blood typing showed them to be MZ; in another four pairs the reverse was true. The differences between mothers' treatment of twin A and twin B, as rated, were calculated. (These characteristics were rated, it should be noted, before the result of the blood typing was known.) The total of these difference scores for the actual DZ-thought-to-be-MZ pairs was 10.5, and for the actual MZ-thought-to-be-DZ pairs it was 3.5 ($p = 0.029$, one-tailed randomization test). The small numbers must make one hesitate to generalize very confidently, but clearly here mothers

TABLE II. Within-Pair Variances of Parent-Initiated Actions for DZ and MZ Pairs

Variable	Variance within DZ pairs	Variance with MZ pairs	F
	Mother (df 29, 17)		
Command-prohibition	7.586	16.588	0.457
Suggestion	11.845	1.794	6.603
Positive action	13.121	19.853	0.661
Neutral action	46.431	25.500	1.821
	Father (df 23, 15)		
Command-prohibition	7.283	5.133	1.419
Suggestion	4.522	5.200	0.870
Positive action	10.348	13.633	0.759
Neutral action	17.304	20.333	0.851

$p < 0.001$.

differentiated more strongly between actual DZ twins, even though they were thought to be MZ.

The results of these four methods, taken together, lead to the conclusions that: a) Parents do treat MZ twins more alike than DZ twins in some respects, but b) they do not introduce systematically greater similarity of treatment for MZ twins in actions which they initiate themselves and which are not contingent on the child's immediately preceding behavior, and c) the overall greater homogeneity of treatment of MZ twins, where it occurs, is in line with their actual, rather than their perceived, zygosity. In other words, parents respond to, rather than create, differences between the twins. An attack on the twin method on this particular ground, therefore, does not seem justified.

REFERENCES

Haseman JK, Elston RC (1970): The estimation of genetic variance from twin data. Behav Genet 1:11–19.

Jinks JL, Fulker DW (1970): Comparison of the biometrical genetical, MAVA, and classical approaches to the analysis of human behavior. Psychol Bull 73:311–349.

Lytton H (1973): Three approaches to the study of parent-child interaction: ethological, interview and experimental. J Child Psychol Psychiatry 14:1–17.

Lytton H (1974): Comparative yield of three data sources in the study of parent-child interaction. Merrill-Parlmer Q 20:53–64.

Lytton H, Conway D, Sauvé R (1977): The impact of twinship on parent-child interaction. J Pers Soc Psychol 35:97–107.

Lytton H, Martin NG, Eaves LJ (in press): Environmental and genetical causes of variation in ethological aspects of behavior in two-year-old boys. Soc Biol.

Scarr S (1968): Environmental bias in twin studies. Eugen Q 15:34–40.

Genetic Influences on Cross-Situational Consistency

Robert H Dworkin

In his influential analysis of contemporary approaches to understanding personality, Mischel [1968] examined the evidence regarding the extent to which measures of personality traits correlate across different situations. His review of the literature for a number of traits indicated that the cross-situational correlations that have been found are typically low, and therefore contrary to what would be expected if traits were an important source of variance in human behavior. Although Mischel's analysis has been vigorously questioned [eg, Alker, 1972; Block, 1977; Epstein, 1977], it has served to stimulate research that examines situations and individual differences concurrently.

Partly in response to Mischel's [1968] emphasis on the role of situations in personality assessment, several authors have begun to study cross-situational consistency itself as an individual difference variable. This research has investigated whether individuals' behavior may be reliably and meaningfully characterized as consistent or inconsistent across situations. In one such investigation of cross-situational consistency as a dimension of personality, Campus [1974] calculated a measure of the consistency of 17 self-rated needs across 16 Thematic Apperception Test (TAT) cards and examined the correlations of this measure with anxiety, extraversion, and field dependence. In addition, she obtained some evidence that the measure of consistency acted as a moderator variable: with increases in consistency, increases in the correlations of some of the need scores assessed by two different methods were obtained. Similarly, Bem and Allen [1974] found that the cross-situation correlations of friendliness and conscientiousness were greater for high consistency subjects than for low consistency subjects, consistency having been assessed by a simple self-report for

Twin Research: Psychology and Methodology, pages 49—56

friendliness and by a questionnaire-derived measure for conscientiousness. To paraphrase Bem and Allen, the data suggest that it is possible to predict some of the people some of the time.

Snyder [1974; Snyder and Monson, 1975], using a somewhat different approach, has constructed a Self-Monitoring Scale that appears to successfully assess the degree to which individuals regulate their behavior in accord with the situations in which they find themselves. Presumably because of their concern for the situational appropriateness of their behavior, high self-monitoring individuals exhibit greater social conformity and greater variability across situations than low self-monitoring individuals [Snyder and Monson, 1975].

The data reported by Campus [1974], Bem and Allen [1974], and Snyder and Monson [1975] indicate that individuals may differ with respect to the extent to which their behavior is consistent from one situation to the next. However, it is not yet clear to what extent cross-situational consistency, when viewed as a dimension along which individuals differ, is a general trait or is specific to specific traits. The measures of cross-situational consistency that have been reported in the literature reflect both orientations. Some authors [Campus, 1974; Snyder and Monson, 1975] approach cross-situational consistency as a general attribute that is reflected in a wide variety of traits. Others [Bem and Allen, 1974] examine cross-situational consistency with regard to specific traits. For example, Campus investigated the correlates of an overall measure of cross-situational consistency derived from a matrix of 17 needs by 16 situations, whereas Bem and Allen assessed each individual's cross-situational consistency for friendliness and for conscientiousness separately. Whether cross-situational consistency is best viewed as a general characteristic of an individual's behavior or as one that is trait-specific is an issue that has so far not been addressed in the research literature (but see Bem [1972]).

The present study sought to further explore the characteristics of cross-situational consistency viewed as a dimension along which individuals differ by examining genetic influences on different measures of cross-situational consistency and on the covariation among these measures. Three measures of cross-situational consistency were examined: self-reported variability for dominance across 12 situations, and the Snyder [1974] Self-Monitoring Scale. Although the latter scale was originally viewed as a measure of the extent to which individuals monitor their self-presentation out of a concern for social appropriateness [Snyder, 1974], recent research has suggested that the scale can be used to identify "those individuals whose social behavior is relatively consistent across situations and those for whom it is more variable" [Snyder and Monson, 1975, p 642].

METHOD

In 1961 and 1962 Gottesman administered the Minnesota Multiphasic Personality Inventory (MMPI) and California Psychological Inventory (CPI) to a sample of 178 same-sex twin pairs of high school age in the Boston area [Gottesman, 1965, 1966]. Eighty-eight of these twin pairs, now adults with a mean age of 30.2 years (SD = 1.45), participated in the present investigation. Fifty-four pairs were monozygotic (32 female, 22 male) and 34 pairs were dizygotic (19 female, 15 male). A number of these pairs had previously participated in a follow-up study in which the MMPI and CPI were readministered [Dworkin et al, 1976, 1977].

The original twin sample was collected through cooperating school systems, advertisements in neighborhood newspapers, and Mothers of Twins Clubs. Additional sampling and demographic data are reported by Gottesman [1966]. The zygosity of most of the pairs in the original sample was established by extensive blood grouping. For reasons of economy, some pairs who were clearly monzygotic (MZ) or dizygotic (DZ) were not blood typed.

Measures and Procedure

The S-R inventory method, introduced by Endler et al [1962], examines the effects of both different situations and different modes of response on the expression of some personal characteristic. In the study of anxiety, for example, the subject rates the extent to which he manifests several different modes of response (eg, heart beats faster; perspires) in several different situations (eg, being alone in the woods at night; waiting in a dentist's office). Recent research, using a variety of behavioral, psychophysiological, and self-report indices in actual situations, has suggested that self-report situation-specific measures such as these can possess appreciable predictive validity [eg, Geer, 1966; Mellstron et al, 1976].

For the present investigation two S-R inventories were developed. An S-R Inventory of Anxiety was constructed that incorporated situations and modes of response from the published inventories of Ekehammar et al, [1974] and Endler et al [1962]. An S-R Inventory of Dominance was also constructed. In these inventories, for each of 12 situations, the subject rates how characteristic each of 11 modes of response is for him on a one to five scale. For more details about these two inventories, and additional analyses, see Dworkin [1977] and Dworkin and Kihlstrom [in press].

Participants were mailed a questionnaire booklet that included the S-R inventories of anxiety and dominance and Snyder's [1974] Self-Monitoring Scale, which consists of 25 true-false items (copies of the questionnaire booklet are

with no phenotypic correlation. These data, therefore, indicate that there is no genetic or environmental (phenotypic correlation minus genetic covariation) covariation between the Self-Monitoring Scale scores and the variability across the dominance situations and across the anxiety situations. The genetic covariation of 0.40 between the variability across the dominance situations and the variability across the anxiety situations is larger than the corresponding phenotypic correlation (0.29), indicating that the covariation between these two measures is either entirely genetic in origin, or the result of positive genetic covariation and some negative enviornmental covariation. This suggests that a genetic pathway exists that accounts for the phenotypic correlation between the variability across the anxiety situations and the dominance situations. Given the relatively small size of the sample, however, these conclusions must be considered tentative.

DISCUSSION

The data for the three measures of cross-situational consistency indicate that genetic influences can be an important source of variance in cross-situational consistency. Evidence of significant genetic variance was found for the Snyder [1974] Self-Monitoring Scale and the variability across the S-R Inventory of Anxiety situation scales. The variability across the S-R Inventory Dominance situation scales, however, did not exhibit evidence of significant genetic variance. Analyses of the phenotypic correlations and phenotypically standardized genetic covariances among the three measures of cross-situational consistency indicated that, in these data, there is no evidence of genetic or environmental covariation between Self-Monitoring and self-reported cross-situational consistency for anxiety and dominance. The genetic covariation between the latter two measures, however, suggests that there is a genetic pathway for their significant phenotypic correlation.

The presence of genetic influences on two of the measures of cross-situational consistency, but not on the third, and the absence of either genetic or environmental covariation between Self-Monitoring and cross-situational consistency for anxiety and dominance, is consistent with the specificity of measures of cross-situational consistency for particular traits. The genetic covariation between the situational variability for anxiety and dominance may be evidence of a more general component of cross-situational consistency shared by these two different traits or evidence of a response style. If the former, this result would provide some support for approaches that view cross-situational consistency as a general attribute that can be reflected in diverse traits. However, consistent support for this position was not found in this study. Considering all the data, the results suggest that cross-situational consistency in personality is best considered with regard to specific traits and behaviors and not as a general characteristic of an individual's behavior.

ACKNOWLEDGMENTS

This research was supported in part by an NSF grant for Improving Doctoral Dissertation Research in the Social Sciences and an NIMH Graduate Traineeship to the author. I thank Andrea L Megela and Barbara W Burke for their encouragement, advice, and assistance, and Irving I Gottesman for making available the twin sample used in this research.

REFERENCES

Alker HA (1972): Is personality situationally specific or intrapsychically consistent? J Pers 40:1–16.

Bem DJ (1972): Constructing cross-situational consistencies in behavior: Some thoughts on Alker's critique of Mischel. J Pers 40:17–26.

Bem DJ, Allen A (1974): On predicting some of the people some of the time: The search for cross-situational consistencies in behavior. Psychol Rev 81:506–520.

Block J (1977): Advancing the psychology of personality: Paradigmatic shift or improving the quality of research? In Magnusson D, Endler NS (eds): "Personality at the Crossroads: Current Issues in Interactional Psychology." Hillsdale, New Jersey: Erlbaum.

Campus N (1974): Transituational consistency as a dimension of personality. J Pers Soc Psychol 29:593–600.

Dworkin RH (1977): Genetic and environmental influences on person-situation interactions. Paper presented at the meeting of the Behavior Genetics Association, Louisville, Kentucky.

Dworkin RH, Burke BW, Maher BA, Gottesman II (1976): A longitudinal study of the genetics of personality. J Pers Soc Psychol 34:510–518.

Dworkin RH, Burke BW, Maher BA, Gottesman II (1977): Genetic influences on the organization and development of personality. Dev Psychol 13:164–165.

Dworkin RH, Kihlstrom JF (in press): An S-R Inventory of Dominance for research on the nature of person-situation interactions. J Pers.

Ekehammar B, Magnusson D, Ricklander L (1974): An interactionist approach to the study of anxiety: An analysis of an S-R inventory applied to an adolescent sample. Scand J Psychol 15:4–14.

Endler NS, Hunt JMcV, Rosenstein AJ (1962): An S-R Inventory of Anxiousness. Psychol Monogr 76(17, Whole No. 536).

Epstein S (1977): Traits are alive and well. In Magnusson D, Endler NS (eds): "Personality at the Crossroads: Current Issues in Interactional Psychology." Hillsdale, New Jersey: Erlbaum.

Geer J (1966): Fear and autonomic arousal. J Abnorm Psychol 71:253–255.

Gottesman II (1965): Personality and natural selection. In Vandenberg SG (ed): "Methods and Goals in Human Behavior Genetics." New York: Academic Press.

Gottesman II (1966): Genetic variance in adaptive personality traits. J Child Psychol Psychiatry 7:199–208.

Haseman JK, Elston RC (1970): The estimation of genetic variance from twin data. Behav Genet 1:11–19.

Mellstrom M Jr, Cicala GA, Zuckerman M (1976): General versus specific trait anxiety measures in the prediction of fear of snakes, heights, and darkness. J Consult Clin Psychol 44:83–91.

Mischel W (1968): "Personality and Assessment." New York: Wiley.

Plomin R, DeFries JC, Rowe DC, Rosenman R (1977): Genetic and environmental influences on human behavior: Multivariate analysis. Paper presented at the meeting of the Behavior Genetics Association, Louisville, Kentucky.

Snyder M (1974): Self-monitoring of expressive behavior. J Pers Soc Psychol 30:526–537.

Snyder M, Monson TC (1975): Persons, situations, and the control of social behavior. J Pers Soc Psychol 32:637–644.

Hemispheric Asymmetry of Function in Twins

Sally P Springer and Alan Searleman

Currently there is considerable controversy concerning the role of genetic factors in the determination of handedness. Existing genetic models do not do a very good job of accounting for the distribution of handedness patterns among relatives [Corballis and Beale, 1976; Hudson, 1875; Levy, 1976], and the classic twin study method also fails to provide support for a genetic contribution to handedness [Collins, 1970]. On the other hand, a variety of what may be considered indirect pieces of evidence are consistent with the hypothesis that variation in handedness is attributable to genetic differences [Levy, 1976], and it has been argued that the high incidence of handedness discordance among monozygotic (MZ) twins is due to special factors that have no bearing upon the tenability of genetic models [Nagylaki and Levy, 1973].

The present work sought to determine the possible role of genetic factors in the determination of another, and perhaps more fundamental, lateral asymmetry — the asymmetry in the functional representation of language in the brain. We used the twin study method and will demonstrate that its judicious use *can* provide important information concerning the factors that contribute to the variation in lateral asymmetries observed among individuals.

The dichotic listening test was employed to obtain a behavioral measure of functional asymmetry. This test involved the simultaneous presentation through headphones of two different spoken syllables, one syllable to each ear. The syllables [pa, ta, ka, ba, da, ga] were employed, with the subject required to identify both syllables presented on a trial. A number of investigators have demonstrated that subjects typically identify with greater accuracy syllables presented to the ear contralateral to the hemisphere housing the speech center [Berlin and MacNeill, 1975; Kimura, 1961; Shankweiler and Studdert-Kennedy, 1967]. Thus, right-handed subjects generally show a right ear advantage in this

Twin Research: Psychology and Methodology, pages 57—62

task, reflecting the specialization of the left cerebral hemisphere for speech in most right handers, while left-handed subjects are more diverse in their ear asymmetry scores, reflecting the greater heterogeneity of brain organization believed to exist among left handers. Recent research has also indicated that the dichotic listening test may be sensitive to a continuum of hemispheric asymmetry of function and that it may tap degree as well as direction of functional asymmetry for speech [Shankweiler and Studdert-Kennedy, 1975]. As such, dichotic listening scores permit a finer assessment of a given individual's pattern of cerebral organization. When degree of ear asymmetry is considered, right handers show considerably more variation than is observed when direction only is considered.

The dichotic listening test we administered consisted of 240 pairs of dichotic syllables, with the data scored to determine the number of correctly identified items in each ear. Various measures of the relative advantage of one ear over the other were employed in subsequent analyses, all yielding comparable results. For simplicity, we will report the findings obtained with the phi coefficient. The phi coefficient is the correlation between side of presentation and correct response and can range from -1.00 to $+1.00$, spanning a continuum from an extreme left ear advantage to an extreme right ear advantage, respectively [Kuhn, 1973]. A value of 0 indicates equal performance in the two ears.

To measure overall performance in the dichotic task, we also computed a total correct score for each subject. This measure is simply the total number of items that were correctly identified regardless of ear of presentation. The total correct and phi scores were not correlated with each other ($r = 0.009$), and hence the total correct (TC) score served as an independent, non-laterality-related measure in the dichotic task.

Subjects were 53 MZ and 35 dizygotic (DZ) twin pairs ranging in age from 13 to 37 years. Zygosity was determined by serological analysis in approximately half the pairs, with a questionnaire shown to have high validity employed in the remaining cases [Cohen et al., 1973]. All twins wrote with the right hand and obtained scores within the range typically observed for right handers on a paper and pencil test of handedness [Crovitz and Zener, 1962].

Table I shows the intraclass correlations that were computed for these MZ and DZ pairs on three measures — the scores on the handedness questionnaire,

TABLE I. Intraclass Correlations for Right-Handed Twin Pairs

	Hand	Phi	TC
MZ (N = 53)	+ 0.30	+ 0.32	+ 0.72
DZ (N = 35)	+ 0.31	+ 0.37	+ 0.31

the phi coefficient, and the total correct scores. Neither phi nor the handedness score showed evidence of heritability. The intraclass correlations were not significantly different for MZ and DZ pairs, nor did the differences approach significance. The TC score, however, did show evidence of heritability. The correlations were significantly greater for the MZ pairs (p < 0.01).

Thus when the subject sample is restricted to right handers, we find no evidence for heritability of degree of handedness or direction and degree of ear asymmetry in the dichotic task. However, total correct performance in the dichotic task — a non-laterality-related measure that can be thought of as a measure of auditory acuity — showed substantial heritability.

An additional 27 pairs of twins containing one right-handed and one left-handed member were also tested. Nineteen of the pairs were MZ and 8 were DZ. We realize that this is a very small sample and that our findings in this group are at best suggestive, but we observed an intriguing pattern of results displayed in Table II. The intraclass correlation for the phi measure was −0.34 for the MZ pairs and +0.09 for the DZ pairs. These values, although not significant, suggest that the MZ discordant pairs are more dissimilar in terms of their phi score than DZ pairs. Using total correct as the measure, these results reverse themselves. The MZ correlation is +0.81, while it is +0.16 for DZ. In this case, MZ twins are more similar, a result comparable to that found among the concordant right-handed twins.

Before discussing the implications of these findings as a whole, it is necessary to demonstrate that the twins we studied are typical of the general population in terms of the measures examined. Such data are provided in Table III. This table gives the mean scores for handedness, phi, and total correct for the concordant right-handed and discordant twins, as well as for groups of left- and right-handed singletons. No differences across zygosity were significant for any measure, nor were any comparisons with singletons significant. As expected, left handers showed smaller phi scores than right handers in each group, although the differences were significant only in the MZ group (p < 0.05).

Table IV shows the frequency of the right ear advantage, regardless of magnitude, for all groups. In this case also, no differences across zygosity or comparisons with singletons were significant. Thus, twins of both zygosities appear to be very much

TABLE II. Intraclass Correlations for Twin Pairs Discordant in Handedness

	Phi	TC
MZ (N = 19)	− 0.34	+ 0.81
DZ (N = 8)	+ 0.09	+ 0.16

TABLE III. Mean Scores as a Function of Zygosity and Handedness

			Hand	Phi	TC
MZ	R/R (N = 53)		21.3	0.142	338.9
	R/L (N = 19)	L	54.7	0.018	355.4
		R	20.4	0.120	346.5
DZ	R/R (N = 35)		21.3	0.139	336.5
	R/L (N = 8)	L	50.2	0.032	337.5
		R	20.2	0.145	316.1
Singletons	L (N = 20)		58.8	0.040	361.7
	R (N = 30)		20.6	0.117	335.8

TABLE IV. Right Ear Advantage as a Function of Zygosity and Handedness

			%
MZ	R/R (N = 53)		87
	R/L (N = 19)	L	68
		R	89
DZ	R/R (N = 35)		80
	R/L (N = 8)	L	63
		R	75
Singletons	L (N = 20)		65
	R (N = 30)		80

like singletons with regard to the relationship between handedness and ear asymmetry. These findings are in conflict with those reported by Boklage at the First International Congress of Twin Studies [Boklage, 1974]. Boklage argued that the relationship between hand usage and direction of ear asymmetry was "released" in MZ twins and that the pairings of these two variables is random in this group. The data on which Boklage based this conclusion, however, suffered from the fact that out of the 40 pairs of MZ twins tested, only 9 had a left-handed member. Moreover, five of these self-assessed left handers were included among the right handers for data analysis on the basis of their scores on a comprehensive handedness battery.

The present results obtained with concordant right-handed twins indicate that the variation in degree and direction of hemispheric asymmetry for speech as measured with dichotic listening is not heritable. That variation, especially in terms of degree, is considerable. It is possible that by restricting our sample to right handers, we have eliminated the only source of genetic variation related to ear asymmetry. Hence our data do not address the issue of whether the differences in cerebral organization found as a function of handedness are under genetic control; they do argue, however, that the variation observed among right handers is not genetic in origin.

The results from the twin pairs discordant for handedness showed a tendency for MZ pairs to be less similar in terms of ear asymmetry than DZ pairs. This may be tentatively explained in terms of the hypothesis that the gradients responsible for the development of bilateral symmetry and asymmetry in the developing embryo are disrupted to some extent by the MZ twinning event. Such a mechanism may be responsible for the mirror imaging of certain features such as handedness, hair whorl direction, and finger pattern often observed in pairs of MZ twins [Newman, 1928; Rife, 1933]. The pattern of results observed in the present study suggests that the process of mirror imaging may extend to cerebral organization as well.

REFERENCES

Berlin C, McNeill MR (1975): Dichotic listening. In Lass NJ (ed): "Contemporary Issues in Experimental Phonetics." Springfield, IL: Charles C Thomas.

Boklage C (1974): Embryonic determination of brain programming asymmetry. Presented at the First International Congress of Twin Studies, Rome.

Cohen DJ, Dibble E, Graw J, Pollin W (1973): Separating identical from fraternal twins. Arch Gen Psychiatry 29:465–469.

Collins R (1970): The sound of one paw clapping: An inquiry into the origin of left handedness. In Lindzey G, Thiessen DD (eds): "Contributions to Behavior Genetic Analysis: The Mouse as Prototype." New York: Appleton-Century-Crofts.

Corballis M, Beale I (1976): "The Psychology of Left and Right." Hillsdale NJ: Lawrence Earlbaum Associates.

Crovitz HF, Zener K (1962): A group test for assessing hand and eye dominance. Am J Psychol 73:271–276.

Hudson PTW (1975): The genetics of handedness – a reply to Levy and Nagylaki. Neuropsychologia 13:331–339.

Kimura D (1961): Cerebral dominance and the perception of verbal stimuli. Can J Psychol 15:166–171.

Kuhn GM (1973): The phi coefficient as an index of ear differences in dichotic listening. Cortex 9:450–457.

Levy J (1976): A review of evidence for a genetic component in the determination of handedness. Behav Genet 6:429–453.

Nagylaki T, Levy J (1973): "The Sound of One Paw Clapping" isn't sound. Behav Genet 3:279–292.

Newman HH (1928): Asymmetry reversal or mirror imaging in identical twins. Biol Bull 55:298–315.

Rife DC (1933): Genetic studies of monozygotic twins III. J Hered 24:443–446.

Shankweiler D, Studdert-Kennedy M (1967): Identification of consonants and vowels presented to left and right ears. QJ Exp Psychol 19:59–63.

Shankweiler D, Studdert-Kennedy M (1975): A continuum of lateralization for speech perception? Brain Lang 2:212–225.

Cardiovascular Reactions During Psychiatric Interview in Twins Discordant and Concordant With Respect to Ischemic Heart Disease

U de Faire and T Theorell

INTRODUCTION

Blood pressure elevation during psychologic strain is a well-known phenomenon [Korner, 1971]. Several studies have been devoted to the interplay between changes in circulatory parameters and psychologic strain [Henry, 1975]. In the present study the relationship between these variables and hereditary factors has been investigated.

The questions to be answered were the following: 1) How do peripheral vasoconstriction, heart rate, and force of left ventricle contraction interact in the promotion of blood pressure elevation as a response to psychologic strain? 2) What elements of the responses are inherited biologically?

MATERIAL

The material under consideration derives from the Swedish Twin Registry. It consists of data for 30 male twin pairs — 17 monozygotic (MZ) and 13 dizygotic (DZ) — aged 51–74 (mean 62), and it constitutes a follow-up of twin pairs previously examined in 1967–1968 [Liljefors, 1970]. These pairs had been selected by means of the angina pectoris questionnaire method according to Rose [1962]. Pairs judged to be concordant or discordant with regard to the probable presence of ischemic heart disease (IHD) at the examination in 1967–1968 were invited to a re-examination, which was performed in 1976.

In the ballistocardiographic analysis, data for four subjects were lost due to technical difficulties. In the plethysmographic analysis, data on ten subjects were lost for the same reason.

Twin Research: Psychology and Methodology, pages 63—68

METHODS

Classification of Ischemic Heart Disease (IHD)

Severity of IHD symptoms was recorded by means of clinical history and electrocardiographic recordings at rest and during physical exercise. A five-graded score was used as described by de Faire et al (1978).

It should be pointed out that the participants arrived after 12 hours fasting without having taken any prescribed tablets the morning of the examination.

Psychiatric Interview

The method of inducing psychologic strain was a structured psychiatric interview. This was divided into three periods, each lasting 5–10 minutes. Period I consisted of questions about childhood. The subject was asked to describe both his parents, how he was punished as a child, how he was treated when compared with sibs, etc. Period II consisted of questions about work conditions. The subject was asked to describe what he was doing at work, conflicts with superiors and work mates, feelings of appreciation from superiors, etc. Period III consisted of questions about present family conditions. The subject was asked to describe his relation(s) with spouses, children, and other close relatives, his sex life, etc.

A brief summary of each subject's responses was written immediately after the interview. An independent psychiatrist subsequently rated the "conflict score" (0–2) of each part of the interview separately. Eighteen subjects reported no conflict, whereas the remaining subjects had a total conflict score varying between 1 and 4.

Hemodynamic Variables

All interviews were preceded by a rest period of five minutes. The subject was lying on a ballistocardiographic bed throughout rest and interview periods. After each one of the six periods a recording was made of the following variables: Heart rate, digital plethysmographic amplitude [Hallböök et al, 1970], ballistocardiographic IJ-amplitude [Smith, 1973], and blood pressure. For all measures except blood pressure the calculation was made from means of ten consecutive heartbeats at the start of each recording. The following measures were used: 1) Heart rate (beats/min) (mean heart rate from the three consecutive rest periods was used as baseline); 2) IJ amplitude (mm) (the amplitudes were calibrated; each mm corresponded to two milli-g of acceleration); 3) plethysmogram aplitude (mm) (these amplitudes were not calibrated); 4) blood pressure (mm Hg). For each interview period, the relative levels (= ratio between interview measure and mean rest measure) of variables 1–4 were calculated. None of the circulatory variables showed a significant change over the rest periods. Results from the resting periods will therefore be presented as a mean of the three rest periods.

STATISTICS

In the analysis of change over periods, ie, from mean at rest to mean during interview, as well as between start and end of interview, paired two-tailed t tests were used.

Since heart rate, IJ amplitude, and plethysmogram amplitude are interdependent, it was essential to make a combined approach. The relative mean interview/rest ratios of these three variables were used in a multiple regression analysis in order to predict mean change in systolic and diastolic blood pressures, respectively. This analysis was based on those subjects who had technically satisfactory recordings of all variables (n = 46). Intrapair and interpair variances for the different variables were calculated according to Osborn and de George [1959]. The dizygotic/monozygotic intrapair variance ratio (F ratio) was calculated for each variable at rest and during interview, and was tested for statistical significance by means of F distribution [Snedecor and Cochran, 1967].

RESULTS

Table I shows the mean relative changes in all circulatory variables as compared with rest. The relative changes during the first and last periods of the interview are also shown. It is obvious that heart rate was the only variable which did not on average exhibit a relative elevation during the interview.

Figure 1 shows the F ratios during rest and interview, respectively, for the variables heart rate, systolic blood pressure, diastolic blood pressure, and logarithm of serum growth hormone concentration. For absolute plethysmographic measures at rest and during interview, no F ratios were calculated, since the interpair variances of these variables among the DZ pairs were significantly greater than those among

TABLE I. Relative Level † of Five Circulatory Variables

	First part of interview	Last part of interview
Heart rate (n = 60)	100.8 ± 0.5	101.1 ± 0.8
IJ amplitude (n = 56)	107.7 ± 2.8**	107.0 ± 3.0**
Plethysmogram amplitude (n = 46)	117.4 ± 7.1*	116.4 ± 8.3
Systolic blood pressure (n = 60)	107.4 ± 0.7***	109.2 ± 0.8***
Diastolic blood pressure (n = 60)	104.3 ± 0.8***	105.4 ± 0.7

† Relative level = (mean measure at interview/mean measure at rest) × 100.
*p < 0.05 ⎫
**p < 0.01 ⎬ compared with mean measure at rest.
***p < 0.001 ⎭

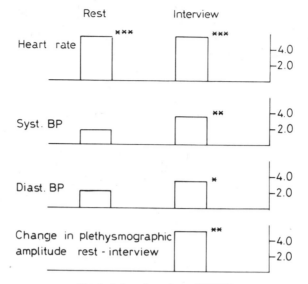

Fig. 1. Intrapair variance DZ/MZ.

the MZ pairs. For relative plethysmographic level during interview as compared with rest ("change"), however, the interpair variances of the DZ and MZ series were similar. Therefore the latter variable but not the absolute level was subjected to intrapair variance analysis. The interpair DZ and MZ variances were similar also for the variables heart rate, blood pressure, and growth hormone. The F analysis indicated genetic influence for heart rate at rest and during interview (both $p < 0.001$), systolic blood pressure during interview ($p < 0.01$), diastolic blood pressure during interview ($p < 0.05$), change in plethysmographic amplitude ($p < 0.01$), and logarithm of serum growth hormone ($p < 0.05$). For blood pressure and serum growth hormone no significant genetic influence was demonstrated at rest.

The multiple regression analysis (Fig 2) yielded a significant ($p < 0.05$) multiple correlation for change in systolic blood pressure only. A great rise could be predicted on the basis of a great rise in heart rate and a decrease in plethysmographic amplitude. A great elevation in diastolic blood pressure was associated ($p < 0.05$) with a decrease in plethysmographic amplitude.

DISCUSSION

The present study indicates that nearly all subjects react to a psychiatric interview with increased systolic and disastolic blood pressure. Heart rate, force of

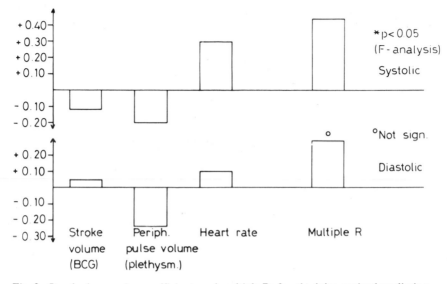

Fig. 2. Standard regression coefficients and multiple Rs for obtaining optimal prediction of change in blood pressure.

left ventricle contraction, and peripheral pulse volume also increase in most subjects. In the interplay between these factors, a large increase in heart rate and a small increase or decrease in peripheral pulse volume are the main determinants of a large increase in systolic blood pressure. A small increase or decrease in peripheral pulse volume is the main determinant of a large increase in diastolic blood pressure.

The analysis of genetic influence showed an interesting difference between the observations made at rest and those during psychologic strain: At rest, only heart rate showed a significantly lower intrapair variance among monozygotic pairs than among dizygotic pairs. During psychologic strain, however, heart rate, systolic and diastolic blood pressure, and logarithm of serum growth hormone were all under significant genetic influence, as judged from the intrapair variances. Furthermore, the relative change in plethysmographic amplitude was under significant genetic influence.

When the subjects in the study were exposed to provocative interviews, some of them showed no visible psychologic reactions, while others reacted vigorously in several ways. The degree and kind of psychologic reaction is probably influenced by genetic factors, and this may partly explain why genetic influence was more easily observable during the stress situation than at rest. It should be mentioned that psychologic "impulsivity" was also observed to be under significant genetic influence in the present study. The number and kind of conflicts reported within MZ pairs did not show more intrapair similarity than those reported within DZ pairs. It should be pointed out that the members of all twin (MZ and DZ) pairs had been brought up together at least until the age of 15. There was no difference in this respect between the MZ and the DZ series. It has been argued that the environment during childhood could be assumed to be more equal for the two members of a MZ pair than for the two members of a DZ pair. A recent review [Plomin et al, 1976] has concluded that most studies comparing similarities in personality traits in members of MZ pairs brought up together and apart demonstrate that being brought up together as compared with being brought up apart does *not* produce more similar personality characteristics in two monozygotic twins. This may support our conclusion.

The ballistocardiographic IJ amplitude reflects the acceleration of flow in the aorta [Smith, 1973]. This dimension has not been corrected for weight, height, and age, which are of significance. However, change in IJ amplitude is still correlated with change in flow acceleration. The fact that the change in flow acceleration was more accentuated among those with more advanced illness signs and symptoms than among others and the fact that change in IJ amplitude was not genetically influenced speaks in favor of the opinion that the ballistocardiographic IJ amplitude is more significantly influenced by the functional state of the myocardium than by genetic factors.

REFERENCES

de Faire et al (1978): Serum pre-beta-1 lipoprotein fraction in twins concordant and discordant for ischemic heart disease. These proceedings, Part C "Clinical Studies."

Hallböök T, Månsson B, Nilsén R (1970): A strain-gauge plethysmograph with electrical calibration. Scand J Clin Lab Invest 25:413.

Henry JP (1975): The induction of acute and chronic cardiovascular disease in animals by psychosocial stimulation. Int J Psychiatry Med 6:145.

Korner PI (1971): Integrative neural cardiovascular control. Physiol Rev 51:312.

Liljefors I (1970): Coronary heart disease in male twins. Hereditary and environmental factors in concordant and discordant pairs. Acta Med Scand (Suppl) 188:511.

Osborn RH, de George FV (1959): "Genetic Basis of Morphological Variation." Cambridge: Harvard University Press, pp 15–24.

Plomin R, Willerman L, Loehlin JC (1976): Resemblance in appearance and the equal environments assumption in twin studies of personality traits. Behav Genet 6:43.

Rose G (1962): The diagnosis of ischaemic heart pain and intermittent claudication in field surveys. Bull WHO 27:645.

Smith NT (1973): Ballistocardiography. In Weissler AM (ed): "Noninvasive Cardiology." New York: Grune & Stratton, Chap 2.

Snedecor GW, Cochran WG (1967): "Statistical Methods." 6th ed. Iowa City: Iowa State University Press.

Identical Twins Reared Apart and Other Routes to the Same Destination

John C Loehlin

INTRODUCTION

My title is "Identical twins reared apart and other routes to the same destination." Let me be clear first as to the "destination" I have in mind. It is estimating
the relative importance of genetic and environmental influences in accounting for
variation in intelligence. We know that people differ in their genes. We know that
people differ in their environments. We believe (or most of us do) that each
person's intelligence is entirely a product of his or her genes and his or her environment. Thus, the differences among people must be a result of differences in their
environments, differences in their genes, or differences in the particular combinations in which these have occurred. And a reasonable and natural first question to
ask, I maintain, is: How much of each? Are the differences in intelligence that
we observe very much a matter of genetic differences among people and very
little a matter of environmental differences? Or exactly the reverse: Does the
environment account for the lion's share of the variation, and the genes for but
little? Or is it about 50—50? Or are particular combinations of heredity and
environment so unique and unpredictable in their effects that knowledge of
either a person's heredity or environment by itself would be of little or no
predictive value? (In technical terms, this would be described as a large heredity-
environment interaction component.) Finally, if favorable heredity and environment tend to occur together in the population (or for that matter unfavorable
heredity and environment), a person's intelligence will to some degree be
predictable from either. If the person who has more favorable genes tends also to
have had a more favorable environment, which would you credit for his high
intelligence? A certain amount of the controversy between hereditarians and

Twin Research: Psychology and Methodology, pages 69—77

environmentalists arises from a tendency of each side to give itself the benefit of the doubt in this matter: Each pounces on the joint variation with cries of "It's mine." (This joint component is, of course, what is technically referred to as heredity-environment covariance or correlation.) So long as we are simply describing conditions in an existing population, it is quite proper to slap the hereditarians' and environmentalists' tiny hands and say, "it belongs to both of you, and if you can't share nicely neither of you gets to play." But there is an important sense in which the controversy about the joint variation is real, significant, and even politically important, and that is when one is predicting what will happen to the joint component when circumstances change. Then the question of what causal structure underlies the joint component of variation is by no means a trivial one. I feel obliged to point out in this connection that it might be nice to know for sure that a substantial gene-environment correlation component actually exists before investing a really heavy amount of passion in fighting over it, but history and experience suggest that this is not a very critical consideration to the more combatively inclined.

So, I submit, if one is interested in some particular human trait, such as intelligence, on which people vary widely, a sensible and interesting first thing to do is to try to split up the variation at least roughly into components associated with genetic variation, with environmental variation, and with the interaction and correlation between these. I said, sensible and interesting *first* thing to do. Once you have grasped the general lay of the land, you will doubtless want to explore further. You might become a specialist in the genetic side, looking at *how* genes affect intelligence (if that is the trait of interest). Do they have their effects primarily on local neural features like rate of forming connections or speed of transmission, or the molecular structure of transmitter substances? Or do they operate at a higher level in the organization of broad brain systems underlying information storage and retrieval? Alternatively, you might become a specialist on the environmental side, in the proper sequencing of experiences, the provision of effective intellectual aids, the role of motivational factors, and the like. Or you might want to look into the interaction between these two domains, or the mechanisms underlying their correlation. Who explores which of these areas is, of course, partly a matter of accidents of training and taste. But the amount of resources society puts into each of these research domains presumably bears some relation to the expected payoff — which rests mainly on two factors. One is the likelihood of success in elucidating the main causal factors in the domain. The other is what we're talking about: the proportion of variation the domain accounts for. Thus, estimating genetic and environmental variance components is a pretty good place to start in considering any given trait, even though it would not be a sensible place to stop.

To wind up the preliminaries, what is this "intelligence" of which I speak? I don't really want to fuss today with definitions, which I have attempted elsewhere [Loehlin et al, 1975]. If we're talking about empirical knowledge, we must start with the intelligence we can measure, ie, with the outcome of some form of intelligence test or rating. Most of what we have to go on in the literature are so-called IQ tests, or measures of the general level of intellectual performance to age. As a theoretician, I wish we had more studies using more differentiated measures such as verbal comprehension, spatial ability, numerical reasoning, and the like. But to a practical man or to a statistician looking at the sizes of the correlations among measures of special abilities in a broad population, general intelligence as measured by the typical "IQ test" is not at all a bad place to start (see, for example, NcNemar, [1964]). (Because some people are touchy on this subject, I should hasten to add that I am not hereby taking a stand on the merits or demerits of IQ testing in the public schools. That question involves many considerations that I haven't the slightest intention of getting into on this occasion.)

IDENTICAL TWINS REARED APART

So, we want to apportion the variation of IQ scores into components. How do we go about it? Ideally, we would like to find people who do not differ in genes but do differ in environmental histories, or people whose environments have been identical but whose genes differ. In practice we can make do with less clear-cut cases, so long as our groups provide us with at least some distinction between degrees of genetic and of environmental resemblance. But the enduring conceptual appeal of identical twins reared apart is that they literally fill the requirements of the first ideal case mentioned above: genetically identical pairs of individuals who have been subjected to different environmental histories. Indeed if we were fortunate enough to have a large sample of identical twins who had been reared in environments differing as much as environments do in the population at large, we could use the covariance between them as a direct estimate of the genetic variance in the population, and the extent of differences between them as an estimate of the combined effects of environment and gene-environment interaction. Finally, the difference between the IQ variance in identical twins reared apart and the population would tell us about gene-environment correlation: If heredity and environment are positively correlated in families in the general population, this will contribute to the total variance of IQ, but in identical twin pairs reared in unrelated families this correlation disappears, and the corresponding decrease in variance gives us a measure of the effect of the covariation in families in general. (I might mention for the benefit of those of you who may have looked at a recent paper by Bob Plomin, John DeFries and me that this refers only to that aspect of gene-environment correlation referred to as "passive" in that paper [Plomin et al, 1977].)

However, we have never had and presumably never will have available a large sample of human monozygotic twins who have been reared from conception on in environments differing to the same degree as do those of members of the population at large. Any inferences from the existing studies of identical twins reared apart must be tempered by this fact. And thus it is essential also to consider other sources of data that can be used in partitioning IQ variance into genetic and environmental components. The two most popular have been the comparison of identical and fraternal twins reared together, and studies involving adopted children.

TWINS AND ADOPTIONS

There have been plenty of ordinary twin studies on general intelligence. One recent tabulation with which I am especially familiar [Loehlin and Nichols, 1976, Tables 4–10] lists 19 studies involving altogether some 6,000 pairs of twins. The average correlation over these studies was about 0.85 for identical twins and 0.60 for fraternals, which suggests a substantial but not overwhelming effect of the genes on intelligence, given the kinds of assumptions usually made in analyzing such data. But critics of the twin method are apt to protest vigrously at these assumptions — particularly the one that the effective environments of fraternal twins are as similar as those of identical twins. Bob Nichols and I looked into the data of the National Merit Twin Study from this perspective [Loehlin and Nichols, 1976, chapter 5]. This large questionnaire study involved 850 sets of late adolescent twins for whom scores were available on a measure of general intellectual performance, the National Merit Scholarship Qualifying Test. Parental reports were obtained on many aspects of the twins' early environments: Whether they were dressed alike as children, whether they were usually in the same classes in school, how much they played together, whether the parents tried to treat them alike or differently and so on. And indeed we found, as nearly everybody else has found who has investigated this point, that identical twins are indeed treated more alike — they are dressed alike more often, are more often together in school, play together more, and so forth. But we went on to ask a second question which is often overlooked: Does this greater similarity of treatment in fact account for the greater similarity of performance on the test? The answer to this question can be obtained by looking *within* the group of identical twins. Some identical twins are dressed alike and some are not, and some are usually kept together in school classes and others are separated. If identical twins who are dressed differently or separated in school are as similar in their test performance as those who are not, it hardly makes sense to attribute the greater test score differences of fraternal pairs to their greater differences on these same environmental variables. And this in fact was the result we obtained: essentially zero correlations for the identical twin pairs between how differently they were treated and how differently they performed on the test. We also didn't find much evidence in our data that the identical twins were, as individuals, much different

from the fraternal twins, or either of these from nontwin individuals, thus
tending to weaken the force of another argument sometimes raised by critics of
the twin method.

I'm going to be very brief on the topic of adoption studies. This is difficult for
me to do, because Joe Horn, Lee Willerman, and I are just winding up a large-
scale adoption study at the University of Texas. We are busy analyzing intelligence
and personality data on members of 300 families who have adopted one or
more children from a private agency that places the children of unwed mothers.
We also have similar test data from the agency files on the unwed mothers. Some
40% of the adoptive families also contain natural children of the adoptive parents.
So you can see we have a wealth of interesting possible comparisons we can make.
We have reported some preliminary findings from our study at various profes-
sional meetings, but there are still a few basic matters that have to be checked
on before we are ready to come to any final conclusions on the IQ data. All I can
say at this point is that from what I have seen in our data so far, I'm not going
out of my way these days to insult either environmentalists or hereditarians!
Also, Dr. Scarr has some further discussion of adoption studies in her contributions to this symposium.

COMBINED ANALYSES

In any case, I want to wind up my comments by examining another strategy
that has much to commend it, certainly in principle. And that is, the strategy of
looking simultaneously at the data from separated identical twins, identical and
fraternal twins, and members of adoptive and ordinary families. R. B. Cattell
pioneered this notion in the 1950s with what he called his Multiple Abstract
Variance Analysis [Cattell, 1953, 1960]. Since the late 1960s the Birmingham
groups of Jinks, Fulker, Eaves, and their colleagues have developed the idea of
expressing family correlations or covariances as a series of simultaneous equations
to be solved by the methods of ordinary or weighted least squares [Jinks and
Fulker, 1970; Eaves, 1969, 1970, 1975; Eaves et al, 1977]. In his 1972 book
Inequality [Jencks et al, 1972], Christopher Jencks carried out an extensive
analysis of twin, adoptive, and ordinary family correlations by the method of
path analysis; the geneticist Sewall Wright actually tried out this technique on
Barbara Burk's IQ data some 40 years earlier [Wright, 1931]. Finally, during
the last few years Morton, Rao, and their colleagues at Hawaii have presented in
a series of papers fairly elaborate path-analysis models which they have applied
to IQ and other data [Morton, 1974; Rao and Morton, 1974; Rao, Morton,
and Yee, 1974, 1976; Rao, MacLean, Morton, and Yee, 1975].

What conclusions have followed from analyzing the data on IQ in this way?
Unfortunately, sometimes rather divergent ones. An interesting comparison is
provided by Jenck's summary correlations for IQ in the US. These data have

been analyzed by Jencks himself [Jencks et al, 1972], by Jinks and Eaves [Jinks and Eaves, 1974; Eaves, 1975], and by Rao, Morton, and Yee [1974, 1976]. If you look at the published outcomes of these different analyses, you are likely to be a bit bewildered. Jencks arrives at a substantial value for gene-environment correlation; Jinks and Eaves find none. Rao et al find heritability to be lower by a factor of 3 among adults than among children; Jinks and Eaves obtain an equally good fit to the data assuming equal heritability in both generations. The Birmingham group find a large component due to genetic dominance; in Honolulu the genes are strictly additive.

What's going on?

I'd like to pursue this question in a bit of detail with respect to two of the analyses: that of the Birmingham group, in papers by Jinks and Eaves [1974], and by Eaves [1975], and that of the Hawaii group in two papers by Rao et al [1974, 1976].

Well, there are some minor differences in the actual data analyzed — for example, Eaves and Jinks use correlations corrected for measurement error and range restriction, while Rao et al employ the uncorrected correlations. Furthermore, these authors make slightly different selections of the data from unrelated children reared together, and Eaves and Jinks do not use some of the equations involving environmental indices that Rao et al do. But these differences prove to be inessential — one can apply both analyses to a common set of correlations and the contrasts between the results remain as striking before.

Nor does the issue appear to be differences in mathematical methods. Actually the underlying mathematical logic of the two approaches should be entirely equivalent. To verify this I carried out the Jinks-Eaves analysis as a path analysis as well as with their original equations and (after correcting a couple of typographical errors in their published equations) obtained identical results. The implementation of the solutions differs in some details between Birmingham and Hawaii: Rao et al fit z-transformed correlations, while Eaves and Jinks work with ordinary correlations, and the two use somewhat different computer algorithms to solve their equations. But these differences are inessential, also. For example, I repeated the Eaves-Jinks analysis, fitting z-transforms and using a different solution procedure, and still obtained the essential features of their results.

If it's not the analytic methods or the data, it must be differences in the assumptions made by the authors. And indeed it turns out to be.

Which assumptions?

Several points can be identified at which the two analyses differ materially in their assumptions.

1. Birmingham assumed the parent and child generations to be alike; Hawaii assumed they might differ.

2. Hawaii assumed the genetic variance to be all additive; Birmingham allowed for possible effects of genetic dominance.

3. Birmingham assumed phenotypic assortative mating, ie, that the correlation between spouses in IQ is due to marriage choices based on the characteristics of the spouse (rather than, say, his or her family background). Hawaii assumed something closer to the latter.

4. Birmingham assumed that the environmental effects common to parent and child were equal to those common to sibs. They also assumed no gene-environment covariance and no direct environmental effect of parents' IQ on child's IQ. Hawaii did not require these as assumptions, although they were allowed as possibilities, and in fact some of the Hawaii analyses did assume the latter two conditions.

5. Finally, the Hawaii analysis incorporated what would seem to be an erroneous equation for identical twins reared apart. It used the genetic parameter appropriate for children, but since the empirical correlation was from the Newman, Freeman, and Holzinger [1937] study, most of whose twins were adult when tested, the genetic parameter for adults should presumably have been used. Note that this will make a difference only if heritability differs between adults and children, but this is what Rao et al concluded to be the case. (I might mention that Arthur Goldberger [1977] has recently pointed out some additional problems in the Hawaii equations and their solutions.)

In most respects, the Hawaii equations are the more general, in that they include the Birmingham assumptions as special cases — except for the assumptions regarding assortative mating and genetic dominance. In another paper [Rao, MacLean, Morton and Yee, 1975] Rao et al state that they have added the possibility of genetic dominance to their equations, but they do not say whether they have reanalyzed the Jencks IQ data with their new equations.

Well, I have; and I can tell you what happens.

First, if you add a dominance parameter to the Rao equations and place other restrictions on these equations corresponding to the Birmingham assumptions, you get essentially the Birmingham results — a satisfactory fit to the data with fewer free parameters than Rao et al require for their equivalently good fits. In particular, Rao et al found that specifying similar values for genetic and environmental parameters in both generations yielded a very poor fit to the empirical correlations; with the inclusion of genetic dominance in the equations this is no longer the case. In other words, at least for these data, the original finding by Rao et al of IQ heritability in adults less than one-third as great as that in children disappears completely if genetic dominance is allowed into their equations. This is true whether or not one incorporates into the model the Birmingham assumptions regarding assortative mating; however, if one doesn't do this, the solution then turns out to be bizarre in other respects. The assumptions regarding dominance and assortative mating thus both contribute to the difference between the Hawaii and the Birmingham results.

Does this mean that the Birmingham solution should be accepted as the optimal one for these data? Not necessarily. For one thing, the Birmingham assumptions of phenotypic assortative mating, parent-child environmental correlation, and no genotype-environment covariation are rather uneasy bedfellows. For another, the selective placement of adopted children is assumed absent in their model, but is probably present in the real world. For still another, different special assumptions about sib and twin environments can be and have been made [Jencks et al, 1972]. Nevertheless, the Birmingham equations do represent one rather economical and straightforward interpretation of the Jencks correlations. And on this model the broad-sense heritability of IQ (according to my solution based on the Birmingham assumptions) is 0.68. That is, roughly 70% of the IQ variation is genetic.

How does this compare with the estimates from the studies of identical twins reared apart? There are four major studies [Jensen, 1970]. Excluding Burt's as in some dispute, the IQ correlations in these studies are 0.78, 0.68 and 0.67. The unweighted mean of these figures is 0.71 and their median is 0.68. As I mentioned, these values can also be taken as estimates, of sorts, of the broad heritability of IQ. I said at the beginning, didn't I, that I was going to be discussing identical twins reared apart — and other routes to the same destination?

REFERENCES

Cattell RB (1953): Research designs in psychological genetics with special reference to the multiple variance analysis method. Am J Hum Genet 5:76–93.

Cattell RB (1960): The Multiple Abstract Variance Analysis equations and solutions: for nature-nurture research on continuous variables. Psychol Rev 67:353–372.

Eaves LJ (1969): The genetic analysis of continuous variation: A comparison of experimental designs applicable to human data. Br J Math Stat Psychol 22 (Part 2):131–147.

Eaves LJ (1970): The genetic analysis of continuous variation: A comparison of experimental designs applicable to human data. II. Estimation of heritability and comparison of environmental components. Br J Math Stat Psychol 23 (Part 2):189–198.

Eaves LJ (1975): Testing models for variation in intelligence. Heredity 34:132–136.

Eaves LJ, Last K, Martin NG, Jinks JL (1977): A progressive approach to non-additivity and genotype-environmental covariance in the analysis of human differences. Br J Math Stat Psychol 30:1–42.

Goldberger AS (1977): "The Non-Resolution of Inheritance by Path Analysis." (mimeo). Madison: Social Systems Research Institute, University of Wisconsin.

Jencks C, Smith M, Acland H, Bane MJ, Cohen D, Gintis H, Heyns B, Michaelson S (1972): "Inequality: A Reassessment of the Effect of Family and Schooling in America." New York: Basic Books.

Jensen AR (1970): IQ's of identical twins reared apart. Behav Genet 1:133–148.

Jinks JL, Eaves LJ (1974): IQ and inequality. Nature 248:287–289.

Jinks JL, Fulker DW (1970): Comparison of the biometrical genetical, MAVA, and classical approaches to the analysis of human behavior. Psychol Bull 75:311–349.

Loehlin JC, Lindzey G, Spuhler JN (1975): "Race Differences in Intelligence." San Francisco: Freeman.

Loehlin JC, Nichols RC (1976): "Heredity, Environment, and Personality." Austin: University of Texas Press.

McNemar Q (1964): Lost: Our intelligence? Why? Am Psychol 19:871–882.

Morton NE (1974): Analysis of family resemblance. I. Introduction. Am J Hum Genet 26:318–330.

Newman HH, Freeman FN, Holzinger KJ: "Twins: A Study of Heredity and Environment." Chicago: University of Chicago Press.

Plomin R, DeFries JC, Loehlin JC (1977): Genotype-environment interaction and correlation in the analysis of human behavior. Psychol Bull 84:309–322.

Rao DC, MacLean CJ, Morton NE, Yee S (1975): Analysis of family resemblance. V. Height and weight in northeastern Brazil. Am J Hum Genet 27:509–520.

Rao DC, Morton NE (1974): Path analysis of family resemblance in the presence of gene-environment interaction. Am J Hum Genet 26:767–772.

Rao DC, Morton NE, Yee S (1974): Analysis of family resemblance. II. A linear model for familial correlation. Am J Hum Genet 26:331–359.

Rao DC, Morton NE, Yee S (1976): Resolution of cultural and biological inheritance by path analysis. Am J Hum Genet 28:228–242.

Wright S (1931): Statistical methods in biology. J Am Stat Assoc 26:155–163.

MZA Twins: Their Use and Abuse

James Shields

FROM NEWMAN TO BURT — A DECLINE?

In 1965 a bright young Maudsley Hospital resident — he has since become a Professor of Psychiatry — was given by Sir Aubrey Lewis the task of criticizing at a Journal Club meeting Dr. Juel-Nielsen's [1965] very fine study of identical twins reared apart (MZAs), which had then just appeared. He began by praising the classical prewar work by Newman, Freeman and Holzinger [1937], a model of its kind. He conceded that my recent study [Shields, 1962] had some merits, but it did not match up to that of Newman et al in its expertise and fine-grained analysis. I've forgotten his objections to Juel-Nielsen's work — perhaps the lack of a control group was one — but the general picture he painted was one of a still further decline from the high standards set by Newman and his colleagues. It is far from my intention to rank the studies in order of merit. Indeed, I would prefer to stress the value of a variety of approaches to the study of twins; and, as I have said, I personally have a high regard for the quality of Juel-Nielsen's work. Nevertheless, I think that if our Maudsley resident had been given the same task a year later on the publication of Sir Cyril Burt's [1966] paper, he could, with some justification, have found that study inferior to its predecessors, despite its greater number of pairs.

Its most obvious limitations were: firstly, its restriction to intelligence and a consequent neglect of other aspects of behavior; and secondly, the lack of information provided about the environments and life histories of the twins. If it were a frequent occurrence for genetically identical twins to be brought up apart, it would be entirely justifiable to concentrate on just one particular aspect of cognitive ability. But the scarcity and value of such material for many branches of psychology and medicine obliges the investigator of twins brought up apart to cast his net more widely, even at the risk of covering some areas relatively superficially. To a varying extent, Newman, Juel-Nielsen, and I have reported on aspects of the twins' personality, social behavior and medical histories, as well as

Twin Research: Psychology and Methodology, pages 79—93

on their intelligence. While we all provided case histories describing the different homes in which the twins were brought up, Burt provided very scanty information in his 1966 paper — he did not even give their ages. However, according to such details as he did give, there was, very surprisingly and contrary to experience, no correlation between the twins in parental occupational class. Upper social class parents had not infrequently farmed out one twin to families in the lowest socio-economic bracket, keeping the other. Similarly upper social class families not infrequently adopted children from the poorest backgrounds. There were more pairs than one would expect with big social-class differences between the parents who brought up the twins. The correlation between social backgrounds was only 0.03. In Conway's [1958] paper, however, before the addition of the final nine pairs to Burt's [1966] sample, there had been a modest correlation of 0.26.

THE BIOMETRIC AND CASE HISTORY APPROACHES

There are two principal uses to which MZA data can be put: biometric analysis and case history analysis. Background information is required whether one is using MZA and other kinship data in order to partition the population variance of a trait into different components, as in the biometric approach, or to investigate, by means of the case history approach, the similarities and differences found between twins of the same genotype when exposed to different environments of a particular kind. Twins are separated for reasons such as illegitimacy, the death of the mother, financial hardship, or unusual circumstances of one kind or another. This makes it unlikely that they are representative of the population; and it is hardly to be expected that they would be placed into different homes at random, as the ideal experiment would require. Such facts need to be borne in mind in the biometric approach, so that one can form some idea of the extent to which MZAs are better for the purpose in hand than MZTs (reared together).

Of course, there is no reason why the two approaches should not be combined. This would normally require teamwork; but if there ever was someone who could have applied them both himself, that was Sir Cyril Burt. It is unfortunate that he did not do so.

BURT: BRILLIANT PIONEER, LIMITED RESEARCH SCIENTIST

Burt was a British pioneer in the development of tests of educational achievement and intellectual potential. As Chief Psychologist to the London County Council from 1913 to 1921, he studied family and social influences on childhood behavior. His book on "The Young Delinquent" [4th edition, 1952], which he is said to have begun writing as long ago as 1905, and his classic on "The Subnormal Mind," recently reprinted [Burt, 1977], show that he had a nose for clinical detail and the development of individual psychopathology; and he had a positive attitude to the treatment of behavioral and scholastic problems. His aim was that every child — including the bright child from a deprived background — should have the most suitable kind of education. In the 1940s he regretted that 40% of those whose abilities were of university standard failed to reach the university. As is better known, he was a pioneer of factor analysis and of the application of R.A. Fisher's methods to the genetic analysis of IQ data. On the vexatious question of heritability Burt [1958] himself put it very clearly when he said that to "an omnibus inquiry," what is the relative influence on a trait of heredity as opposed to environment, "there can be no single answer. We can only try to determine, for this or that type of environment, for this or that population, and for this or that type of assessment, how far the observable results appear to be influenced by each of the two main groups of factors."

Despite his achievements, many of those sympathetic, as well as those hostile, to his approach and conclusions about genetics had reservations about his work as a research scientist. Jensen [1974] noted "puzzling discrepancies and ambiguities" in his data. In the controversy that raged in the correspondence columns of the London *Times* last year, Burt's biographer, Professor L.S. Hearnshaw, [*The Times,* November 13, 1976] acknowledged that there were "legitimate suspicions as to some of his data on twins;" and colleagues told how he wrote spoof letters to the British Journal of Statistical Psychology which he edited. Papers published as written jointly or even solely by collaborators, such as Miss Conway and Miss Howard, were said by his secretary to have been solely Burt's work and written when he was no longer in touch with them. This does not mean he invented his data — or his colleagues. Even if it is best to discount Burt's data, if only because of the careless, casual, and cavalier way it was presented, his conclusions may not be incorrect. The planting of the Piltdown skull did not disprove the theory of evolution. Other workers have confirmed Burt's findings such as an MZA correlation of 0.77 on group tests of intelligence and a lower correlation with respect to educational achievement.

AUTHOR'S ONLY CONTACTS WITH BURT

I have been asked to say something about my personal connections with Burt. That is easy. I never met him. Nor did Eliot Slater, my former chief; and we did not exchange reprints. But we did have some communication.

The first time was in 1963, when a manic-depressive twin (MZT) admitted to the Maudsley Hospital said that she and her sister were tested — it was said for Cyril Burt — when they were about 10, in 1930.* We thought it worth trying to discover whether their childhood IQ tests were still available. Burt's successor at University College advised me to telephone him at home, which I did. Courteously, Burt

*From what the twins now (1977) say, it seems that they were not tested for Burt but at the London School of Economics for Herrman and Hogben (1933).

regretted he no longer had any records of twins from that period — which was per-haps not altogether surprising. The twins' own recollection is of being tested by "two dear ladies," aged about 28 or 29, they thought. That would put them in their late 70s now. One was tall, slim, blonde and elegant; the other "didn't register." Whether these were the elusive Misses Conway and Howard, we have no way of knowing.

The second occasion when I spoke to Burt was in 1969, after requesting per-mission to reproduce a table from one of his publications. I still have the old man's elegantly hand-written reply, giving me leave to make use of his table, and adding some "trifling suggestions" of further tables I might use from his own work, instead of other people's. In thanking him, I took the opportunity to ask him on the telephone if he could supply any further details about the backgrounds of his MZA twins. Miss Conway would have had that information, he said; but she had emigrated to "Australia, New Zealand, or somewhere" — and that was that.

DID BURT ABUSE THE MZA METHOD?

In his 1966 paper Burt indicated that identical twins were brought up apart more frequently than I had surmised; but I must confess I was curious to know how he had so easily been able to raise his total by nine pairs between 1958 and 1966, long after Miss Conway had emigrated. It now seems that in 1958 Burt him-self most probably wrote the paper attributed to Miss Conway, his collaborator in the 1930s. One might think there was a certain amount of one-upmanship as to whether Burt or I had studied more MZAs (Table I). In recent years, since Jensen [1974] and Kamin [1974] have drawn attention to the way Burt sometimes allotted IQ scores to parents and other relations on the basis of interview informa-tion rather than tests, the ungenerous thought crossed my mind that the reason for his not giving raw scores but only IQ assessments for his MZAs might be that some had not been tested. Admittedly, that is contrary to what Burt says in his 1966

TABLE I. Number of Pairs of Separate MZ Twins in Successive Reports of the Studies of Burt and of Shields

Author, year	Number of pairs
Burt, 1943	15
Burt, 1955	21
Shields, 1956	38
"Conway," 1958	42
Shields, 1962	44
Burt, 1966	53

paper. However that may be, there is little point in further tarnishing Burt's reputation — or, for that matter, whitewashing it. (I must admit to a sneaking sympathy with his assessments: It is not so very different from what some of us do in the assessement of personality and even psychiatric diagnosis! Rating techniques are frequently used by experimental psychologists to provide a quantitative score.) But if Burt did not test some of the twins, he should have said so. Unfortunately in Burt's case we shall never know. Among the papers destroyed at his death were test sheets with names and ages of children and various calculations thought by his secretary to have been used by Burt for his published papers on twins. They may well have included data on the twins themselves. Ironically, these papers were destroyed on the advice, not of Burt's pupils, but of two social scientists who had no sympathy for his views about genetics.

In describing his work on MZA twins, Burt seems to have been more interested in dotting the i's and crossing the t's of his analysis of variance approach to family IQ data than in presenting a research report. Jensen [1974] has said it seems as if he "regarded the actual data as merely an incidental backdrop for illustration of the theoretical issues," and from his personal knowledge of Burt Eysenck [1977] believes this may be true. Burt never presented his MZA findings adequately. There are many uncertainties about how and when (and perhaps even whether) the twins were tested, and what their scores were. The lack of supporting case-history-type information is surprising in view of Burt's own emphasis on assessment rather than score, and the sensitivity he showed earlier for the effect of environmental influences interacting with temperament in the development of childhood psychopathology and school failure. So much for Burt for the time being.

KAMIN ACCUSES SHIELDS OF INVESTIGATOR BIAS

If Burt may have abused the MZA method by his restrictive approach and uncertain data, Kamin [1974] has abused the whole genetic approach to intelligence. He finds fatal flaws of one kind or another (usually another!) in the different MZA studies. Since there was no evidence in my study of the age effect he claims to have detected in the work of Newman and Juel-Nielsen, he alleges instead that investigator bias, unconscious or conscious, influenced my administration and scoring of the intelligence tests. Investigator bias is hard to refute, but I shall do my best and, if I may, present some further analysis of my own study.

Admittedly, in my evaluation of personality similarities and differences, I took advantage of having talked to both twins myself, often seeing them together. I unashamedly presented my subjective impressions and, so far as I could, the objective evidence on which they were based. I am only too aware of the hazards of unreliability and investigator bias here. But as regards the intelligence tests, I find it difficult to see how I could have seriously influenced the results of pencil-and-paper tests for which there are only right or wrong answers. In the Vocabulary test, only the Synonyms section of the Mill Hill scale was used. Here the subject has to underline which out of six words means the same as the word printed above them in larger type. The possibility of accepting or rejecting a dubious definition simply did not arise.

In my statistical analysis I took the opposite line from Burt and used the raw scores, even if I did not think they were the best estimate of a subject's intellectual potential; but I commented on cases where I thought the test unsuitable, and looked for the most likely reasons for the larger differences between twins. The only exception was to reject as invalid a score of only 1 in the 48-item Dominoes test, on the grounds that the subject could not have understood the instructions. I rejected three such cases altogether in the separated and control groups. The score of one MZA female twin could further be seen to be invalid because she had entered the figures 7 and 8 on her answer sheet, ignoring the instruction that only numbers up to 6 could be entered in the blank domino. Though she did a little less well than her sister in the Vocabulary test, it was clear she was not mentally retarded. In her case the Dominoes test was administered when I was ill by a colleague who had no experience with these tests. If her Dominoes score of 1 were counted, these twins would have differed by 38 points on the combined test — a much bigger difference than in any other pair. Kamin, however, included it, using the 38-point difference as the biggest support for his argument that the pairs where I tested both twins were significantly — and suspiciously — more alike than the few pairs where I did not test them both. Since in this pair one twin was brought up by an unrelated friend of the family, it also entered into Kamin's analysis which claimed large differences in intelligence in twins not brought up by members of the same family, as several of my pairs had been.

INDEPENDENT RETESTING

Last month we were able to examine these twins again (Sf3) after 22 years. They were tested on the WAIS by different clinical psychologists, blind as to the previous test results and the controversy surrounding them. On the basis of the previous tests, I predicted that the twin who failed the Dominoes test would have an IQ of about 90 and her sister a higher one of about 100. The results were that the first twin's Full Scale IQ was 92, so she was clearly not an imbecile or moron as implied by Kamin. The IQ of the second twin was 111. After being tested, the first twin said she could remember not understanding the Dominoes instruction 22 years ago but she had not liked to ask for further clarification.

There is independent evidence of IQ in the Scandinavian twin tested by me (Sf19). She too was given the WAIS and she secured a better score than she had on the Dominoes test in which I thought she had not done herself justice. However, I would like to stress that I did not "adjust" her Dominoes and Mill Hill scores in order to make her more like her South American sister, but accepted the original large difference of 24 points at face value. To turn to a pair where I tested both twins, I found the MZA schizophrenic twins (Sm P4) both to be of dull intelligence, with a 7-point difference on the combined test. Independent evidence from psychologists in different hospitals reported Wechsler IQs of 75 and 76!

So much for alleged investigator bias making the twins more alike than they really were. Other aspects of Kamin's criticism have been well dealt with by two of today's symposiasts, Drs. Sandra Scarr-Scalapatek [1976] and John Loehlin [Loehlin et al, 1975], and, in devastating detail, by Dr. David Fulker [1975]. I would not have been surprised by finding that twins brought up by different members of the same family were more alike than pairs in which one or both twins had a nonfamilial placement; I thought it might well be so [Shields, 1962, p 100] with respect to intelligence tests. I shall deal with that and other similar points next.

MZAs WITH MOST AND LEAST SIMILAR ENVIRONMENTS

As I made clear in my book, many of the MZA twins I studied were brought up by relatives, and some were separated rather late or reunited in childhood. Obviously some pairs had early environments that were considerably more alike than others, but all were worth studying nonetheless. Even when the twins were brought up by different relatives, the respective families differed considerably in the age and personality of the parents, the presence of other children, financial circumstances, a town or country environment, the emotional climate of the home, and so on. When a pair spent holidays together, the twin in the strange home would sometimes cry to go back to her "own" mother. On average, the environments were less alike than those of identical twins reared in the same home. They would be more like those of cousins, and cousins are less alike in IQ than twins.

In a further attempt to evaluate the influence of shared family environments, I have been comparing the MZAs who had the least and the most different environments. Before comparing these two groups with respect to intelligence, I "purified" the material by removing pairs where the tests may have been unsuitable for estimating IQ or where there were other confounding factors such as neurological disease that might interfere with the assessment of the effects of ordinary family differences. The "purification" excluded a) children (8 and 14 years old) for whom the Dominoes test was unsuitable; b) those whose first language was Welsh, Danish, or Spanish (though all spoke English too), for whom the Mill Hill Vocabulary test was unsuitable; c) a pair of schizophrenics obtained from the Maudsley Psychiatric Twin Register; and d) pairs where one or both twins had congenital syphilis, epilepsy, or disseminated sclerosis. Eight pairs were excluded in this manner, some for more than one reason.

To obtain the purified group with the *most* similar environments I picked those where the twins had at some time gone to the same school and who had also been reared by relatives (Table II). Three of these were late separations (not until the

TABLE II. Subdivision of Shields' [1962] Separated
MZ Twins

Subgroup criteria	Number of pairs
Most similar environments ("purified")	16
Brought up by close relatives and	
went to same school (10 pairs were	
separated late or reunited)	
Least similar environments ("purified")	12
Separated by 18 months	
Not reunited in childhood	
Never at same school	
Not reared by mother and MGM	
"Other"	10
Excluded in "purification" (8)	
Late separated, reared in	
institutional homes (2)	
Total pairs tested	38
(Dominoes and Mill Hill)	

twins were 7, 8, or 9 years old), and in seven pairs the twins were reunited before leaving school — not always very happily, it may be said. As a group these may be thought to have had relatively similar family and educational experiences and more mutual contact than the other MZAs.

To obtain a purified group with the *least* similar environments, I stipulated that the twins should have been separated before the age of 18 months. (Seven of these were said to have been separated at birth and a further three at 6 months.) Furthermore, they should not have been reunited in childhood or have ever attended the same school. The 12 pairs found in this way included none where one twin was brought up by the mother, the other by the maternal grandmother. In five of them the twins were reared by parents who were unrelated to one another.

I shall compare these two groups with each other and also with the remaining ten. These "others" include the eight pairs excluded in the "purification" and two pairs which did not meet the criteria of the two groups just described: these two pairs were separated relatively late and brought up in different institutional homes. The group includes the four pairs where I was unable to test both twins because one or both were in Scotland, Germany, or South America.

Table II shows the resemblance found in the three MZA subgroups, in the total of 38 MZAs tested, and in the 34 matched MZT controls, or identical twins brought up together. The findings are in respect of the combined nonverbal Dominoes and Mill Hill Vocabulary tests.

A brief word about the tests: The Mill Hill Vocabulary scale is a well established test designed for use in conjunction with the highly reputed Raven's Matrices. The nonverbal Dominoes test is not so well known, but it correlates highly with the Matrices. It was used recently on twins in Brazil [Telles da Silva et al., 1975] with results comparable with mine. I combined the two, in an empirical fashion, to form a single estimate of intelligence.

I should point out that the mean difference between the twins shown in Table III is not a difference in conventional IQ points, but it may not be so very far from that. The raw test scores are not easy to transform into accurate IQ equivalents, with a mean of 100 and standard deviation of 15. Arthur Jensen [1970], and our chairman, Irving Gottesman [1968], have each tried their hand at it, with differing results. Jensen's attempt has been criticized as minimizing IQ differences, while Gottesman's produces bigger differences and, to my mind, a misleadingly large proportion of mentally retarded twins in the sample. But it so happens that the mean raw score difference comes half-way between the IQ differences as calculated by Jensen and Gottesman, so it may not be too misleading if one forgets that they are not IQ differences. Table III also shows the intrapair correlation between the twins. The correlations would not be affected by IQ transformation.

Comparing the purified MZAs with the most and least similar environments, it is surprising that the former twins (r = 0.87) are only marginally more alike than the latter (r = 0.84). This lends little support to the view that partially shared family and educational environment is responsible in the main for the intellectual resemblance found in the separated twins in my study. But if we look at the individual scores and case histories in the "most similar" group we find that in two of the pairs with the largest differences — 25 and 12 points, respectively — the twin who did more poorly in the tests is said to have been "nearly given up for dead" at birth. In the first of these he was also described as "black and blue" and his test score was low. (The other possibly birth-injured twin's score was about IQ 100.) If we omit these two pairs, the correlation for the remaining 14 rises to 0.92 and the mean difference drops to only 5.12 points compared with one of

TABLE III. Monozygotic Twins (data of Shields [1962])

Composite intelligence test (Dominoes and Mill Hill Vocabulary)	N	Mean difference (points)	Within-pair correlation
Reared apart			
Most similar environments	16	6.81	0.87
Least similar environments	12	8.21	0.84
Others (not "purified")	10	14.8	0.47
Total	38	9.40	0.78
Reared together (controls)	34	7.38	0.76

8.21 points in the "least similar" group. This may suggest a modest influence of family environment. It is, however, suprising that resemblance in the admittedly "nonpurified" control group was less close than that in the purified separated twins. Lest we try to make too much out of these correlations, it must be pointed out that they are not significantly different from one another on these numbers.

You might wonder why I did not remove the birth-injured twins in my present zeal for purification, along with the epileptics and others. I found it difficult to draw a sharp line between pathological and other perinatal hazards of twins. If, like Munsinger [1977], I had excluded all those with possible birth difficulty or with moderate differences in birthweight, or where one twin was described as "weakly" as a child, on the grounds that they might be instances of the placental "transfusion syndrome" in MZ twins, there would have been very few pairs left. Information about condition at birth was not available in many of the MZAs.

Turning to the 12 pairs with least similar environments, there were, as I said five where the twins were reared by unrelated parents. In one of these they were both adopted and did not meet until they were investigated at the age of 36 years; one of them had not even known she had a twin. This pair had a 5-point difference. These five pairs were no less alike in intelligence (mean difference 8.0 points) than the remaining seven brought up within the same family network (difference 8.4), bearing out what I was saying about family environment.

Three pairs in this group with the least similar environment had large test differences of 16, 17, and 20 points. In the pair with 17 points difference, social and educational influences were probably important. The brighter of these twins, Jacqueline, was brought up by her paternal uncle who ran a family business and sent her to an independent grammar school. Beryl's adoptive father — the husband of a distant maternal cousin — was a "ne'er-do-well" who from time to time ran an amusement arcade. She had an ordinary elementary school education. I shall return to the question of socioeconomic class later. The reasons for the other two big differences in this group are unfortunately obscure. It is of interest that the twins in this group were also surprisingly similar in extraversion on the personality questionnaire ($r = 0.91$), averagely alike in neuroticism ($r = 0.38$), and strikingly alike in my assessment of personality based on life history data and observations on interview.

THE IMPORTANCE OF INDIVIDUAL ENVIRONMENT

As we can see from Table III, it is in the group of ten "others" that we find the biggest differences in intelligence, the mean difference being 14.8 points and the correlation 0.47. It is a heterogeneous group. Though in only two pairs were the twins brought up by related parents, there were five late separations. When we compare their intelligence test results, we find 8-year-old twin girls, both adopted, with identical scores; and in four other pairs there were average differences of 7 to 10 points. The other five pairs, however, showed large differences of 14 to 30 points, and they included four where neuropsychiatric illness such as epilepsy or disseminated sclerosis probably contributed to the difference. To complicate the picture, in two of these five pairs with big differences, the colleagues who tested one twin for me were inexperienced in administering tests of this kind – in one case English was not the first language of either the twin or the colleague.

This analysis points to the apparently great importance, in my sample at least, of idiosyncratic factors peculiar to the individual. Such factors may have more influence on intelligence test performance than shared family environment in general or the kind of environmental similarity often experienced by MZTs in particular. It points to the importance of E_1 rather than E_2, to use the terminology of the Birmingham school about which Lindon Eaves has been telling us today. Birth injury and physical illness were perhaps the most obvious examples, but the idiosyncratic factors need not be physical and may include test-taking attitude. Above all, the findings confirm the substantial influence of genetic factors. Family environments can vary quite a lot without obscuring the basic similarity in a pair of genetically identical twins, though it must also be remembered that even monozygotic (MZ) twins reared together can differ quite widely [Shields, 1962].

SOCIOECONOMIC CLASS: HOW MUCH SELECTIVE PLACEMENT?

I now come to the question of socioeconomic class. Despite Burt's peculiar sample which I mentioned earlier, it is not very realistic to expect MZA twins to be adopted into families at random. If social class influences intelligence, biometric analysis of MZA data may have to make allowance for selective placement.

In my book I tried to indicate the extent of the differences in parental occupation. In one pair the biological father, an unstable ship's carpenter in a Scandinavian country, kept one twin and sold the other to a successful doctor in South America to settle his debts (Sf19). Such a difference is exceptional. Large differences were rare, but several moderate differences in the fathers' occupations were observed. These included foreman-tailor versus quarryman, master-baker versus agricultural laborer, clerk versus horse-and-cart man, and carpenter (with his own business) versus jobbing gardener. In my previous analysis [Shields, 1962] I found no very remarkable tendency for the twin brought up in a home of lower socioeconomic standing to have the lower intelligence. This was so in only 10 out of the 17 pairs where the twins differed in both these respects.

The customary division of occupations, on which I mainly relied, into the Registrar-General's five social classes, with Social Class III accounting for about half the population, is of limited value. The more recent Hope-Goldthorpe social grading of occupations [Goldthorpe and Hope, 1974] offers a more finely graded scale. With a colleague, John Hewitt, we have been trying out this scale. Our very provisional results show that a wide range of father's occupation is represented in the MZAs. The within-pair difference in the social standing of the fathers may have been about half as great as it would have been had the twins been placed at random. Within pairs, the correlation between fathers' social class difference and the twins' difference in intelligence was about 0.25 for the purified part of the sample. This indeed is close to the 0.29 reported by Burt [1966]. Perhaps only a small correction to MZA IQ correlations in intelligence may be required to allow for the effects of selective placement. However, our provisional findings, based on small numbers, must be treated with caution. Of interest is the observation that female MZA twins tended to marry men who were alike in social status: Their husbands' occupational scores had a correlation of 0.46.

USES OF THE CASE HISTORY APPROACH

I hope I have indicated some of the ways in which case history information can be used. Even single pairs can be of interest for observing the effect on behavior of particular environmental factors, and the ways in which twins may resemble one another despite these differences. In the recent "Encyclopaedic Handbook of Psychological Medicine" [Krauss, 1976] the entry on Heredity refers to the "unusual insight into the effects of genotype" provided by the Newman, Shields, and Juel-Nielsen MZA monographs. "The best way to read these books," it is said, "is to keep them by the bedside and read about one pair of twins every night."

In pair Sf8 [Shields, 1962], Olive and Madge were separated seven days after birth because their mother was too ill to look after them both. Madge, the stronger was taken by a childless paternal aunt, while the mother kept Olive. The twins, when I saw them, had not met since the age of 3 years, when the mother had wanted Madge back. But the aunt insisted on keeping her and prevented the twins from meeting. Olive was brought up knowing she had a twin, and always longed to meet her. Madge was not told she had a twin till she was 9 years old, and then went in fear of being kidnapped. These learned attitudes still colored their views about each other when I saw them at the age of 35. Olive wanted me to persuade Madge to see her, while Madge made it a condition that I would never attempt to do so.

Though Madge was sent to a private school and Olive missed much schooling on account of poor health, they differed by only 3 points on the intelligence tests; and on the personality questionnaire both were relatively low in extraversion and high on neuroticism. Although they were seen in their own homes, they both remained standing for a few minutes at the beginning of the interview. I was impressed by the very similar way in which they spoke about their shyness, their liking for sport, and their taste in music. One mentioned Tchaikovsky's first piano concerto as one of her favorite works, the other

Rachmaninof's second. Olive said she liked Handel's "Messiah" best of all. Madge was a piano teacher. On top of her pile of music when I visited was a copy of "The Messiah." (Admittedly "The Messiah" is rather well known, and it would have been even more remarkable if it had been Handel's "Israel in Egypt.") Since the twins had never communicated with one another, the question of collusion did not arise.

In view of their fondness for music I arranged for Dr. Rosamund Shuter [1966] to give them both Wing's standardized test of musicality. Madge's score placed her among the top 10% of the population. Olive, who had no musical training, was also above average, coming between the top 20 and 30%.

The history of this pair illustrates what is so often said about the importance of heredity, environment, and their interaction. But it also shows much detailed resemblance in behavior of a kind that it would have been natural to ascribe to mutual influence, had the twins been brought up together.

By far the most extensive case history of a single set of multiple MZ births, incorporating the results of detailed psychological investigations, is not a pair of separated twins, but the study by Rosenthal and colleagues [1963] of the Genain quadruplets, all of them schizophrenic, but differing in their experiences within the same family and in the severity of their illnesses. MZA studies are in one respect an extension of the study of differences in MZTs designed to detect the influence of environment. MZA studies, however, are prospective, in the sense that they examine the later effect of known differences in environment. This is in contrast to the retrospective search for environmental causes in pairs known to be discordant for a clinical condition such as schizophrenia.

The case history approach is not inconsistent with biometric genetic analysis. Jinks and Fulker [1970] were able to analyze my data. Gottesman and I attempted both in our Maudsley schizophrenic twin study [Gottesman and Shields, 1972]. It is remarkable that among the few authors I can recall as having quoted any of the case histories of my MZA study are the mathematical population geneticists Cavalli-Sforza and Bodmer [1971]. They cited a pair of twin boys (Sml) who were surprisingly alike and both free from behavior problems, although one was reared by a mentally ill mother; and another male pair (SmP9) in which the twin who probably suffered malnutrition in infancy and was harshly treated by his stepmother was later hospitalized with the diagnosis "hysteria in an inadequate psychopath." (He was one of those who could not grasp the Dominoes instructions and scored only 1; but both twins had the same poor Vocabulary score.)

MZAs AS VALIDATION OF MZT/DZT METHOD

A further use of MZAs should be mentioned, though this has been implicit in much of what I have already said. They can be used to test the hypothesis that MZTs are more alike than DZTs on account of the more similar within-family environment of the MZTs. This is one of the most frequent criticisms of the classical twin method. For this purpose it is no disadvantage that the environments of the two twins may not differ very much. Indeed, it would be best if the MZA twins were exposed to environments as similar in as many respects as possible, except for having different rearing parents and no close mutual contact. Perhaps the strongest conclusion to be drawn from MZA studies so far — those of personality and schizophrenia as well as of IQ — is that MZ twins do not have to be brought up in the same subtly similar family environment for them to be alike.

CONCLUSIONS

I have tried to indicate some of the many uses of twins brought up apart and to deal with some of the abuse which MZA studies have recently attracted. I focused mainly on the case history approach and on my own study.

It is a pity that Sir Cyril Burt's study was restricted to intelligence. It may be prudent to disregard his work in the future on account of the many uncertainties about his data and the casual way in which he presented his findings. If so, we are still left with 75 pairs presented in much greater detail — warts and all — by Newman et al. In the United States (19 pairs), Shields in the United Kingdom (44 pairs) and Juel-Nielsen in Denmark (12 pairs), and a number of single case reports besides (eg, Burks and Rose, 1949]. Burt's pairs were children, Newman's mostly young adults, Shields's somewhat older, and Juel-Nielsen's mostly elderly. (Eight of his pairs had the advantage of being ascertained through the Danish Twin Register, then limited to twins born between 1870 and 1910.) Such conclusions as one can draw concerning the inheritance of intelligence will not be much altered by the omission of Burt's MZA data, since his within-pair correlations were not significantly higher than those of the others.

The need to take stock after writing off Burt — or at least putting him on the shelf — draws attention to what would have been desirable in any case: the need to replenish. Twins brought up apart will probably remain unusual, unless social conditions in Japan are such that it is still quite normal there for twins to be separated. I hope I have made clear that there are merits in studying partially separated pairs as well as those in which the twins have been exposed to moderate or extreme differences in environment. But surely it should one day be possible to collect a further sample and, without neglecting the lessons learned from earlier studies, to improve upon them and test new hypotheses concerning intelligence, personality and mental illness. I doubt if MZAs will ever be numerous and representative enough to provide the main evidence about environment, or about genetics, but they furnish critical examples of persons of identical genotype reared in different homes. They can give unique real-life illustrations of some of the many possible pathways from genes to human behavior — and so will always be of human and scientific interest.

REFERENCES

Burks BS, Roe A (1949): Studies of identical twins reared apart. Psychol Monogr 63:1–62..

Burt C (1943): Ability and income. Br J Educ Psychol 13:83–98.

Burt C (1952): "The Young Delinquent," 4th Ed. London: University of London Press.

Burt C (1955): The evidence for the concept of intelligence. Br J Educ Psychol 15:158–177.

Burt C (1958): The inheritance of mental ability. Am Psychol 13:1–15.

Burt C (1966): The genetic determination of differences in intelligence: A study of monozygotic twins reared together and apart. Br J Psychol 57:137–153.

Burt C (1977): "The Subnormal Mind." 3rd Ed, reissued. London: Oxford University Press.

Cavalli-Sforza LL, Bodmer WF (1971): "The Genetics of Human Populations." San Francisco: WH Freeman.

Conway J (1958): The inheritance of intelligence and its social implications. Br J Stat Psyschol 11:171–190.

Eysenck HJ (1977): Burt C: Foreword to "The Subnormal Mind." 3rd Ed, reissued. London: Oxford University Press, pp v–xvii.

Fulker DW (1975): Review of "The Science and Politics of IQ" by LJ Kamin. Am J Psychol 88:505 537.

Goldthorpe JH, Hope K (1974): "The Social Grading of Occupations." Oxford: Clarendon Press.

Gottesman II (1968): Biogenetics of race and class. In Deutsch M, Katz I, Jensen AR (eds): "Social Class, Race, and Psychological Development." New York: Holt, Rinehart and Winston, pp 11–51.

Gottesman II, Shields J (1972): "Schizophrenia and Genetics: A Twin Study Vantage Point." New York: Academic Press.

Herrman L, Hogben L (1933): The intellectual resemblance of twins, Proc Roy Soc Edin 53:105–129.

Jensen AR (1970): IQs of identical twins reared apart. Behav Genet 1:133–148.

Jensen AR (1974): Kinship correlations reported by Sir Cyril Burt. Behav Genet 4:1–28.

Jinks JL, Fulker DW (1970): A comparison of the biometrical genetical, MAVA and classical approaches to the analysis of human behavior. Psychol Bull 73:311–349.

Juel-Nielsen N (1965): Individual and environment. A psychiatric-psychological investigation of monozygotic twins reared apart. Acta Psychiatr Scand Suppl 183.

Kamin LJ (1974): "The Science and Politics of IQ." New York: Wiley.

Krauss S (ed) (1976): "Encyclopaedic Handbook of Medical Psychology." London:Butterworths.

Loehlin JC, Lindzey G, Spuhler JN (1975): "Race Differences in Intelligence." San Francisco: WH Freeman.

Munsinger H (1977): The identical-twin transfusion syndrome: A source of error in estimating IQ resemblance and heritability. Ann Hum Genet (London) 40:307–321.

Newman HH, Freeman FN, Holzinger KJ (1937): "Twins: A Study of Heredity and Environment." Chicago: University of Chicago Press.

Rosenthal D, et al (1963): "The Genain Quadruplets." New York: Basic Books.

Scarr-Salapatek S (1976): Review of "The Science and Politics of IQ" by LJ Kamin. Contemp Psychol 21:98–99.

Shields J (1956): Twins brought up apart. Paper read at Symposium on Genetics, Maudsley Hospital, October, 1956, and later published [Shields J (1958) Eugen Rev 50:115–123].

Shields J (1962): "Monozygotic Twins Brought up Apart and Brought Up Together." London: Oxford University Press.

Shuter R (1966): Hereditary and environmental factors in musical ability. Eugen Rev 58:149–156.

Telles da Silva BT, Osorio MRL, Borges, Salzano FM (1975): School achievement, intelligence, and personality in twins. Acta Genet Med Gemellol (Roma) 24:213–219.

Development of Piagetian Logicomathematical Concepts: Preliminary Results of a Twin Study

Arleen S Garfinkle and Steven G Vandenberg

INTRODUCTION

A number of twin studies have been done on various cognitive abilities. However, all but one (The Louisville Twin Study [Wilson, 1974, 1976]) have been done on adolescents and adults. All of these studies have used a standard psychometric approach to cognition, which has recently been criticized on the grounds that studies of cognition should have a theoretical framework [DeVries, 1974]. Hence, this is the first behavior genetic study based on Piaget's theory of cognitive development. The purpose of this study is to examine the genetic and environmental influences on the development of Piagetian logicomathematical concepts in young children. The goal is to test 200 same-sex, 4- to 8-year-old Anglo twin pairs from the entire socioeconomic status range.

METHODS

Subjects

Twin pairs were solicited through school districts and mothers-of-twins clubs in the greater Denver-Boulder area. The present sample of 100 twin pairs consisted of 51 MZs, 25 male and 26 female, and 49 DZs, 23 male and 26 female.

Following the precedent of Cohen and associates [1975], zygosity was determined by a mother's questionnaire about twin similarities and differences, phenylthiocarbamide (PTC) tasting, and fingerprinting. Bloodtyping was done on pairs of questionable zygosity.

The twin pairs were relatively equally distributed among 4-, 5-, 6-, and 7-year-old groupings. The mean age was 5 years 10 months, with a standard deviation (SD) of 1 year 1 month.

Twin Research: Psychology and Methodology, pages 95–100

The majority of the present sample was at the higher end of the socioeconomic status distribution. Father's occupation was coded according to the Duncan modification of the National Opinion Research Center (NORC) occupational prestige scale [Reiss, 1961] with a possible range of 20–93. This sample ranged from 41 to 93, with a mean of 73.7, representing a technical worker, and a comparatively small SD of 9.3. Education was coded on an arbitrary scale of 1–16. Father's education ranged from 5 to 16, and mother's from 6 to 16. Father's education mean of 10.5 represented 4 years of college, with a SD of 2.6. Mother's education mean of 9.7 represented 2 years of college, with a SD of 1.7.

Procedure and Description of Measures

Twins were individually administered four cognitive tests: 1) The Piagetian Mathematical Concepts Battery (PMCB) consists of 15 tasks representing the three Piagetian concepts of Conservation, Classification, and Seriation. The PMCB has an α reliability of 0.87 [Garfinkle, Vandenberg, and Simons, 1977a, 1977b]. 2) The Raven Coloured Progressive Matrices (PM) is the child's form (4–11 years) of the well-known adult Progressive Matrices. Among children 6½–12 years old, it has a test-retest reliability of 0.90 [Raven, 1965], and it was included in this study as a measure of reasoning ability. 3) The Peabody Picture Vocabulary Test (PPVT) is also a well-known standardized test, with a form A-form B reliability of 0.77 [Dunn, 1965]. 4) Visual Memory, immediate and delayed (VM), was developed by Vandenberg. It has been used successfully in a number of recent studies, with a split-half reliability of 0.63 for 7- to 18-year-olds [DeFries et al, 1974; Foch, 1975; Zonderman et al, 1977]. However, it has not previously been used on children as young as in this sample.

The parents also filled out two questionnaires which were included as independent measures of the environment. The Attitudes Toward Education Questionnaire is not included in this report. However, the Moos Family Environment Scale (FES) was analyzed. The FES consists of ten subscales: Cohesion, Expressiveness, Conflict, Independence, Achievement Orientation, Intellectual-Cultural Orientation, Active Recreational Orientation, Moral-Religous Orientation, Organization, and Control. Each family received an average standard score for each subscale [Moos, 1974].

RESULTS

Since there were no significant mean or variance sex differences in cognitive performance, all data were pooled across sex for all further analyses. There were also no significant mean or variance differences in performance between the MZ and DZ samples. So, for some data results were determined for the whole sample.

Out of 105 possible, the PMCB mean was 74.9, with a SD of 19.7. Out of 36 possible, the PM mean was 17.7, with a somewhat small SD of 5.4. For the PPVT, the mean was 59.3, out of 150 possible, with a SD of 9.1. Since this test is meant for people up to 18 years old, this mean was not unreasonable. For this analysis, the memory score was the sum of the immediate and delayed memory scores. Of 40 possible, the mean was 12.3, with a SD of 7.8. This indicated that these young children did not do very well on this visual memory task.

As expected, the PMCB had the highest correlation with age: r = 0.78. Next was the PPVT, with r = 0.73. The PM correlated 0.62 with age, while VM correlated 0.44. Because of such high correlations with age, age was partialed out of performance in all further analyses.

For this sample of 200 children, correlations among tests were calculated, after partialing out age. A 0.16 correlation between the PPVT and the PM indicates that these tests do indeed measure separate abilities which are independently yet equally related to performance on the Piagetian battery (both correlate 0.30 with the PMCB, p < 0.01). Yet the 0.30 correlations with the PMCB indicate that the PMCB is itself measuring something other than vocabulary and reasoning ability. Memory is apparently essentially unrelated to the other abilities (mean r = 0.17, p > 0.01). However, this may be due to the lack of test validity for this age group. (Very young children tend to point at the pictures they like, and not necessarily the ones they remember.)

Intraclass Correlations

With age partialed out of test performance, the intraclass correlations were calculated using the residual scores, as seen in Table I. As a check on the sample, the same calculations were done on height and weight (Table I). The intraclass correlations for height and weight were within the range of the expected, and previously reported, values [Wilson, 1976b].

TABLE I. Intraclass Correlations and Between-Pair and Within-Pair Variances for the Cognitive Tests, and Height and Weight

Measure	Intraclass correlation		Between-pair variance		Within-pair variance	
	MZ (51)	DZ (49)	MZ	DZ	MZ	DZ
PMCB	0.62	0.65	85.44	106.24	51.92	57.05
PM	0.44	0.60	6.32	12.36	7.95	8.23
PPVT	0.72	0.61	28.85	21.67	11.08	14.03
VM	0.25	−0.08	11.87	−3.87	36.23	53.40
Height	0.93	0.43				
Weight	0.91	0.53				

For the cognitive tests, there were no significant differences between any of the MZ and DZ intraclass correlations. This fact, and the magnitudes of these correlations (except for Memory), suggest the need to look carefully at the between-pair environmental variance, also presented in Table I. All the MZ-DZ within-pair variance comparisons were in the expected direction. However, some of the between-pair variances were considerably larger than the within-pair variances, and discrepant between MZs and DZs, although not significantly. With such small within-pair variance differences between MZs and DZs, the PMCB and PM reversal of the expected direction of the MZ and DZ intraclass correlations was mainly due to the discrepancy of the between-pair variances.

Environmental Analysis

These results led to the analysis of some of the environmental data. Since there were no significant mean or variance differences in any of the environmental variables between MZs and DZs, the environmental analyses were performed on the whole sample. The environmental variables considered were Father's Occupation, Father's and Mother's Education, and the ten subscales of the FES. With age partialed out, the correlations between the environmental variables and test performances were calculated. For N = 162, the critical value ($p < 0.01$) was r = 0.199. The significant correlations indicated that Father's Occupation (r = 0.21), Mother's Education (r = 0.25). Intellectual-Cultural (r = 0.20) and Moral-Religious (r = 0.22) orientation might influence PMCB performance. Similarly, Moral-Religious orientation might influence PM and Intellectual-Cultural orientation might influence PPVT performance. None of the environmental variables significantly correlated with Memory.

The sample was subjected to stepwise multiple regression analyses to determine the significant environmental influences on performance. The independent variables were the 13 environmental variables, while the dependent variables were performances on the cognitive tests. As the correlations indicated, there were no significant environmental influences on Memory. The significant influences on the other cognitive tests are shown in Table II. These results must be considered tentative, since environmental information was only available for 44 MZ and 37 DZ pairs.

Of course, age explained the major part of the variance in these tests, accounting for 40–61% of the variance in test performance. However, including the environmental variables accounted for 42–65% of the total variance in cognitive performance, which is considerable.

For the PMCB, high Mother's Education level and Moral-Religious orientation also increased PM performance. This Mother's Education effect was also found during the development of the PMCB [Garfinkle, Vandenberg, and Simmons, 1977b]. Moral-Religious orientation also increased PM performance. PPVT performance was increased by Intellectual-Cultural orientation and Conflict within the family. The only significant

TABLE II. Significant Variables in Stepwise Multiple Regressions of Environmental Variables on Cognitive Test Performances*

Test	Variable entered	Significance of F for variable to enter equation	R^2
PMCB			
	Age	< 0.01	0.61
	Mother's Education	< 0.01	0.63
	Moral-Religious	0.01	0.65
PM			
	Age	< 0.01	0.40
	Moral-Religious	< 0.01	0.42
PPVT			
	Age	< 0.01	0.52
	Intellectual-Cultural	< 0.01	0.54
	Conflict	0.01	0.56

*N = 164.

environmental influence which is somewhat difficult to interpret is that of Moral-Religious orientation, for which the authors have no explanation.

DISCUSSION AND CONCLUSIONS

Keeping in mind that only half of the final sample has been analyzed, some tentative conclusions seem obvious. First, although related to the Progressive Matrices and the Peabody Vocabulary Test, the PMCB is evidently measuring something distinct from the abilities measured by the other cognitive tests. Similar results were reported by Klippel in 1975. Further analyses of these test interrelationships will be undertaken when the whole 200-pair sample is available.

Second, the sample was tested during a crucial developmental period. This is illustrated by the fact that there did not appear to be any significant genetic variance in cognitive performance after age was partialed out. This is in contrast to previous reports of significant genetic variance found in adults for the Progressive Matrices and vocabulary tests [DeFries et al, 1976]. However, this is the first behavior genetic study using these measures in this age range, and the first genetic study of the development of mathematical concepts based on Piaget's theory.

Finally, some significant family environmental influences on cognitive performance are emerging. If these environmental effects remain stable with a larger sample, they will give direction to future research on environmental manipulation for the purpose of influencing cognitive development.

ACKNOWLEDGMENTS

This study was supported in part by a grant from the Council on Research and Creative Work, University of Colorado, and in part by a grant from the Spencer Foundation.

REFERENCES

Cohen DJ, Dibble E, Grawe JM, Pollin W (1975): Reliably separating identical from fraternal twins. Arch Gen Psychiatr 32:1371–1375.
DeFries JC, Ashton GC, Johnson RC, Kuse AR, McClearn GE, Mi MP, Rashad MN, Vandenberg SG, Wilson JR (1976): Parent-offspring resemblance for specific cognitive abilities in two ethnic groups. Nature 261:131–133.
DeFries JC, Vandenberg SG, McClearn GE, Kuse AR, Wilson JR, Ashton GC, Johnson RC (1974): Near identity of cognitive structure in two ethnic groups. Science 183:338–339.
DeVries R (1974): Relationships among Piagetian achievement and intelligence assessments. Child Develop 45:746–756.
Dunn LM (1965): "Peabody Picture Vocabulary Test Manual." Circle Pines, Minn: American Guidance Service.
Foch TLT (1975): "Analysis of the Unreduced Battery for the Colorado Family Study of Specific Reading Disability." Unpublished master's thesis, University of Colorado.
Garfinkle AS, Vandenberg SG, Simmons RJ (1977a): Development of a battery of Piagetian logico-mathematical concepts. Behav Genet (Abstract) 7:60.
Garfinkle AS, Vandenberg SG, Simmons RJ (1977b): Development of a battery of Piagetian logico-mathematical tasks. (Submitted for publication.)
Klippel MD (1975): Measurement of intelligence among three New Zealand ethnic groups. J Cross-Cult Psychol 6:365–376.
Moos R (1974): "Family Environment Scale and Preliminary Manual." Palo Alto, California Consulting Psychologists Press.
Raven JC (1965): "Guide to Using the Coloured Progressive Matrices." London: HK Lewis.
Reiss AJ (1961): "Occupations and Social Status." Glencoe, Illinois: Free Press.
Wilson RS (1974): Twins: Mental development in the preschool years. Develop Psychol 10:580–588.
Wilson RS (1976a): Twins and siblings: Concordance for school-age mental development. (Unpublished manuscript.)
Wilson RS (1976b): Concordance in physical growth for monozygotic and dizygotic twins. Ann Hum Biol 3:1–10.
Zonderman AB, Vandenberg SG, Spuhler KP, Fain PR (1977): Assortive mating for cognitive abilities. Behav Genet 7:261–271.

School Achievement and Test Results for Twins and Singletons in Relation to Social Background

Siv Fischbein

INTRODUCTION

Many earlier studies of achievement in twins and singletons of the same age have found that twins tend to score somewhat lower on tests than singletons. This is true for different types of tests but is particularly evident for tests of verbal ability [Husén, 1960; Koch, 1966; Mittler, 1971]. Some researchers, however, have come to the conclusion that the differences between twins and singletons tend to diminish with advancing age and finally disappear [Dales, 1969; Wilson, 1974].

The reason for the frequently observed "twin handicap" is not obvious. It has sometimes been explained by a biological inferiority, caused by a greater vulnerability in twins both during the prenatal period and at birth. Another possible explanation is the special situation experienced by twins. Husén [1960], for instance, pointed out that "the partners within such a group seem to develop other means of communication than linguistic symbols, which are necessary for the establishment of contacts with adults. Gestures, intonation, and similar means are used instead of verbal symbols." It also seems probable that twins have fewer adult contacts, on the average, since these will tend to diminish given a larger number of children in the family.

If environmental factors are of vital importance for the inferiority shown by twins on test results, a difference between socioeconomic groups would be expected, so that the "twin handicap" would be smaller in higher socioeconomic groups, where there is probably more stimulation of mental development. The research results presented in this field so far are contradictory [Zazzo, 1960; Heisterkamp. 1977].

Twin Research: Psychology and Methodology, pages 101–109

MATERIALS AND METHODS

In 1964 a longitudinal study of physical and mental growth in twins and controls of matched age was started (the SLU project [Skolöversty-Relsens och Lärar-Högskolans Utvecklingsstudie — A Growth Study by the Board of Education and the Stockholm School of Education). The results presented in this paper have been collected in the SLU study. The twins were taken from the 40 largest cities and towns in Sweden and their controls were attending the same classes as the twins. Originally the sample consisted of 94 pairs of monozygotic (MZ) twins, 133 dizygotic (DZ) pairs of the same sex, 96 dizygotic (DZ) pairs of opposite sex and 1,194 controls of approximately the same age as the twins.

Several kinds of information have been collected for the twins and their controls: physical measurements (height, weight, etc), achievement and ability test results, behavior ratings, background variables. A more detailed description of the project and the methods used has been given by Ljung, Bergsten-Brucefors, and Lindgren [1974].

A comparison between the twin groups and the group of singletons for physical development has been made by Ljung, Fischbein, and Lindgren [1977]. In this paper achievement test results will be presented for the twin categories (MZ, DZ like-sexed, and DZ unlike-sexed) and for the group of singletons. The twins and their controls were given standardized achievement tests in Swedish (reading and writing) in grade 3 (at approximately 10 years of age) and mathematics in grades 3 and 6 (at approximately 13 years of age). (A description of the standardized tests used in the Swedish school system to equalize marks has been given by Ljung [1965]). At the age of 12, in grade 5, a group-administered intelligence test (DBA) was given to the participants in the SLU project. This test consisted of three parts: a test of verbal ability (opposites), inductive reasoning (letter groups), and clerical speed (similar numbers). A grouping of the twins and controls on the basis of socioeconomic status of their parents has been made in the SLU project. Father's occupational status was classified into three groups: I) employers (mostly university graduates); II) salaried employees (eg, small owners, administrators); III) manual workers. For a further description of the social background variables collected for the SLU material see Lindgren [1976].

A two-way analysis of variance was used to study differences between twins and controls in relation to social background.

RESULTS

Standardized Achievement and DBA Test Results for Different Twin Cateogries

A comparison between different twin categories (MZ, DZ like-sexed, and DZ unlike-sexed) on achievement test results for Swedish and mathematics in grade 3 and for mathematics in grade 6 is presented in Table I. The use of the standardized achievement tests is optional in Swedish schools and as can be seen from

TABLE I. Achievement Test Results for Swedish in Grade 3 and for Math in Grades 3 and 6 for Different Twin Categories

		MZ			DZ (like-sexed)			MZ (unlike-sexed)			df	F
		M	SD	N	M	SD	N	M	SD	N		
Boys												
Grade 3	Swedish	21.1	7.7	53	22.6	8.5	93	20.3	8.8	58	2/202	1.35
	Math	28.1	7.4	53	29.2	9.9	92	28.9	10.4	58	2/202	0.78
Grade 6	Math	41.0	14.2	78	43.3	17.7	106	43.1	17.6	69	2/251	0.45
Girls												
Grade 3	Swedish	22.3	6.8	59	22.0	7.5	83	23.6	8.4	53	2/193	0.85
	Math	22.8	7.6	57	26.0	9.4	83	26.6	9.3	52	2/190	3.02
Grade 6	Math	32.2	12.7	76	36.1	15.3	111	38.5	14.8	70	2/255	3.62*

*$p < 0.05$.

Table I more classes have been taking them in grade 6 than in grade 3. A comparison of the SLU group with a random sample of all Swedish school children has been made by Fischbein [1976]. There is no reason to believe that the SLU sample is biased, since the distributions for the two groups are not significantly different from each other. The results in Table I show very small differences for the twin categories. For girls in grade 6 only there is a significant F value due to MZ twins scoring lower than the other two twin categories on the math test.

The differential ability test (DBA) given to the twins in grade 5 includes, as earlier mentioned, three different tests, measuring verbal, inductive, and clerical speed abilities.

The differences between the twin groups also tend to be very modest for these tests and are not significant for any of the ability tests. The conclusion reached from the comparison of different twin groups (MZ, DZ like-sexed, and DZ unlike-sexed) for results on standardized achievement and the DBA tests is that the differences between twin categories generally are very small and insignificant in these respects. In the following comparisons of test results for twins and controls in relation to social background, the twins will thus be treated as one group.

Standardized Achievement and DBA Test Results for Twins and Controls in Relation to Social Background

As mentioned earlier, a two-way analysis of variance has been used to study differences between twins and controls in relation to socioeconomic status (social groups I, II, and III). This has been done separately for boys and girls. The results on the standardized achievement test in Swedish in grade 3 are shown in Table II. It can be seen from Table II that the F ratio for rows (F_r) is high and significant for girls, while it is very low for boys. This indicates that there is a difference in test results between twin girls and their controls, but not for twin boys in comparison to singletons. The group means (for girls $M_{twins} = 22.5$ and $M_{controls} = 24.3$ and for boys $M_{twins} = 21.6$ and $M_{controls} = 22.0$) clearly show that this is due to a lower average achievement for twin girls in comparison to controls on this test. The F ratio for columns (F_c), on the other hand, is significant for both boys and girls, illustrating that socioeconomic factors are important determinants of test results. As would be expected, both twins and controls from social group I get the highest scores, on the average, and those from social group III the lowest. There is no significant interaction effect (F_i) for either girls or boys, which means that the difference between twin boys and their controls is negligible in all social groups and that the twin girls tend to score lower than singletons irrespective of social background.

Table III reports the variance analysis results for the mathematics test in grade 3. The results for the math test in grade 3 show the same trend as for the test in Swedish. Row effects are significant for girls but not for boys, owing to lower average scores for twin girls in comparison to controls. For both boys and girls the column effects are significant and the interaction effect insignificant. The results for grade 6 correspond with the results in grade 3. There is a significant difference between twin girls and their controls due to the twin girls' lower average achievement. For twin boys the difference is small and insignificant. The F ratios for columns are significant for both boys and girls and the interaction effects are negligible for both sexes. All the achievement tests (Tables II, III) thus show a consistent trend.

TABLE II. Analysis of Variance for the Standardized Achievement Test in Swedish in Grade 3

Source of variation	Sum of squares	Degrees of freedom	Variance estimate	F^a
Boys				
Rows (twins/controls)	22.00	1	$22.00 = S_r^2$	0.37
Columns (social groups)	2,445.25	2	$1,222.62 = S_c^2$	21.00**
Interaction	19.31	2	$9.66 = S_i^2$	0.16
Within cells	21,650.62	372	$58.20 = S_w^2$	
Girls				
Rows (twins/controls)	424.06	1	$424.06 = S_r^2$	8.29**
Columns (social groups)	1,104.87	2	$552.44 = S_c^2$	10.80**
Interaction	48.94	2	$24.47 = S_i^2$	0.047
Within cells	17,333.00	339	$51.13 = S_w^2$	

$^a F_r = S_r^2/S_w^2 \, ; F_c = S_c^2/S_w^2 \, ; F_i = S_i^2/S_w^2.$
**$p < 0.01$.

TABLE III. Analysis of Variance for the Standardized Achievement Test in Math in Grade 3

Source of variation	Sum of squares	Degrees of freedom	Variance estimate	F^a
Boys				
Rows (twins/controls)	27.25	1	$27.25 = S_r^2$	0.16
Columns (social groups)	3,896.44	2	$1,948.22 = S_c^2$	11.95**
Interaction	123.12	2	$61.56 = S_i^2$	0.37
Within cells	41,877.25	257	$162.95 = S_w^2$	
Girls				
Rows (twins/controls)	1,679.50	1	$1,679.50 = S_r^2$	11.14**
Columns (social groups)	2,091.25	2	$1,045.62 = S_c^2$	6.94**
Interaction	227.56	2	$113.78 = S_i^2$	0.75
Within cells	39,318.31	261	$150.64 = S_w^2$	

^{a}Same as Table II.
**$p < 0.01$.

A corresponding analysis of results from the DBA tests for twins and controls by socioeconomic status follows.

Table IV presents the analysis of variance results for the verbal test for boys and girls respectively. The substantial sex difference noted for achievement test results, where twin girls but not twin boys scored significantly lower than their controls, has disappeared for the verbal ability test. Both twin boys and twin girls show significantly lower average scores than their controls, even if the difference still is larger for the girls (for girls $M_{twins} = 4.7$ and $M_{controls} = 5.3$; for boys $M_{twins} = 4.8$ and $M_{controls} = 5.2$). Socioeconomic factors are, as expected, of considerable importance for determining their results on the verbal test. There is no significant interaction effect, which means that twins tend to score lower than controls in all social groups.

Table V illustrates the analysis of variance results for the DBA test measuring inductive ability. The same trend can be seen for the inductive test as for the verbal test. The F ratios for rows and columns are significant for both boys and girls. There is no interaction effect for either sex.

The results for the clerical speed test (Table VI) seem quite different from the other two DBA tests. Social background, for instance, obviously is of little importance for results on the clerical speed test for both boys and girls. The twin boys also seem to get significantly lower scores on this test in comparison to controls. The twin girls, on the other hand, show a similar achievement as their controls. No significant interaction effects are found for either boys or girls.

TABLE IV. Analysis of Variance for the DBA Verbal Test

Source of variation	Sum of squares	Degrees of freedom	Variance estimate	F^a
Boys				
Rows (twins/controls)	19.41	1	$19.41 = S_r^2$	6.12*
Columns (social groups)	332.75	2	$166.37 = S_c^2$	52.48**
Interaction	13.88	2	$6.94 = S_i^2$	2.18
Within cells	1,817.50	573	$3.17 = S_w^2$	
Girls				
Rows (twins/controls)	58.73	1	$58.73 = S_r^2$	18.88**
Columns (social groups)	132.68	2	$66.34 = S_c^2$	21.33**
Interaction	1.68	2	$0.84 = S_i^2$	0.27
Within cells	1,751.64	563	$3.11 = S_w^2$	

[a]Same as Table II.
*p < 0.05.
**p < 0.01.

DISCUSSION

Comparison of achievement test results for twins and controls shows an interesting sex difference. Twin girls tend to score lower, on the average, than their controls, while there is no significant difference for the boys. This inferiority of

TABLE V. Analysis of Variance for the DBA Inductive Test

Source of variation	Sum of squares	Degrees of freedom	Variance estimate	F^a
Boys				
Rows (twins/controls)	18.29	1	$18.29 = S_r^2$	4.54*
Columns (social groups)	86.03	2	$43.02 = S_c^2$	10.70**
Interaction	14.52	2	$7.26 = S_i^2$	1.80
Within cells	2,301.84	572	$4.02 = S_w^2$	
Girls				
Rows (twins/controls)	25.88	1	$25.88 = S_r^2$	7.01**
Columns (social groups)	32.45	2	$16.22 = S_c^2$	4.39*
Interaction	1.04	2	$0.52 = S_i^2$	0.14
Within cells	2,085.52	565	$3.69 = S_w^2$	

[a]Same as Table II.
*$p < 0.05$.
**$p < 0.01$.

TABLE VI. Analysis of Variance for the DBA Clerical Speed Test

Source of variation	Sum of squares	Degrees of freedom	Variance estimate	F^a
Boys				
Rows (twins/controls)	22.27	1	$22.27 = S_r^2$	5.97*
Columns (social groups)	0.09	2	$0.04 = S_c^2$	0.01
Interaction	13.25	2	$6.63 = S_i^2$	1.77
Within cells	2,107.60	565	$3.73 = S_w^2$	
Girls				
Rows (twins/controls)	7.60	1	$7.60 = S_r^2$	1.91
Columns (social groups)	1.38	2	$0.69 = S_c^2$	0.17
Interaction	24.65	2	$12.32 = S_i^2$	3.11
Within cells	2,210.89	558	$3.96 = S_w^2$	

[a]Same as Table II.
*$p < 0.05$.

twin girls in comparison to controls has also been found for physical development: Twin girls tend to be smaller and weigh less during puberty, while no such difference is found for boys (Ljung, Fischbein, and Lindgren [1977]).

There is no obvious explanation of why twin girls are more different from their controls than twin boys. One reason could be a higher mortality for the twin boys, thus an effect of selective survival [Ljung, Fischbein, and Lindgren, 1977]. A comparison of mortality for infants in Sweden from 1926 to 1967 for boys and girls shows that approximately 1% more boys than girls among singletons died in infancy. For the twins, however, the corresponding proportion is a little more than 2% [Official Statistics of Sweden, 1958; Medlund et al, 1977]. The proportion of stillborn children in 1955 was approximately 1% for both boys and girls among singletons. For twins, on the other hand, this proportion was approximately 5 and 3% for urban twin boys and twin girls respectively [Official Statistics of Sweden, 1977]. Thus the sample of surviving twin boys seems to be a more positively selected group than that of the twin girls.

There is no interaction effect between being a twin and socioeconomic status, which means that when there is a "twin handicap," it tends to be of the same magnitude irrespective of social background. This is in agreement with results from some earlier twin studies showing that a more stimulating environment will not have the effect of reducing the "handicap" [Zazzo, 1960; Koch, 1966; Mittler, 1970].

REFERENCES

Dales RJ (1969): Motor and language development of twins during the first three years. J Genetic Psychol 114:263–271.

Fischbein S (1976): "Att vara tvilling" [Being a twin]. (Report No 2). Stockholm: Department of Educational Research, School of Education.

Heisterkamp G (1972): Zur Psychologie der Zwillings-situation. Schule Psychol 19:346–360.

Husén T (1960): Abilities of twins. Scand J Psychol 1:125–135.

Koch HL (1966): "Twins and Twin Relations." Chicago: University of Chicago Press.

Lindgren G (1976): Height, weight, and menarche in Swedish urban school children in relation to socio-economic and regional factors. Ann Hum Biol 3:501–528.

Ljung B-O (1965): "The Adolescent Spurt in Mental Growth." Stockholm: Almqvist och Wiksell.

Ljung B-O, Bergsten-Brucefors A, Lindgren G (1974): The secular trend in physical growth in Sweden. Ann Hum Biol 1:245–256.

Ljung B-O, Fischbein S, Lindgren G (1977): A comparison of growth in twins and singleton controls of matched age followed longitudinally from 10 to 18 years. Ann Hum Biol 4: 405–415.

Medlund P, Cederlöf R, Floderus-Myrhed B, Friberg L, Sörensen S (1977): A New Swedish Twin Registry containing environmental and medical base-line data from about 14,000 same-sexed pairs born 1926–58. Acta Med Scand Suppl 600.

Mittler P (1970): Biological and social aspects of language development in twins. Dev Med Child Neurol 12:741–757.

Mittler P (1971): "The Study of Twins." London: Penguin Books.

Official Statistics of Sweden (SOS) (1958): "Befolkningsrörelsen, År 1955" [Vital statistics, 1955]. Stockholm: Central Bureau of Statistics.

Wilson RS (1974): Twins: Mental development in the preschool years. Dev Psychol 10:580–588.

Zazzo R (1960): "Les Jumeaux; Le Couple et la Personne." Paris: Presses Universitaires de France.

Monozygotic Concordance in a Cognitive Skill (Time Estimation)?

Edward Grant

INTRODUCTION

Attempts to find an organic basis for timing and for the capacity to experience and estimate duration began almost 90 years ago; yet they remain unsuccessful. As a result doubt was cast on the notion that individuals make use of a stable "internal clock" to judge the passage of time. However, the discovery of many "biologic clocks" in nature led to a second look at the psychophysiology of time in humans [eg, Gooddy, 1959; Cohen, 1967].

But for the psychologist, the conceptual gap between the capacity for biologically functional timing on the one hand, and that for the conscious experience of duration and the ability to estimate and compare durations, on the other, is too great to be acceptable, even though it is quite likely that the latter is dependent on the former. Accordingly it seemed wiser to seek first some reasonably unequivocal empirical evidence of physiologic and/or hereditary involvement in a particular aspect of temporal experience, and only afterwards to try to pin down its organic substrate. The capacity to estimate time is an ideal cognitive skill for this purpose, in that it is clearly definable, operationally delimitable, and has been the subject of numerous previous investigations not only dealing with the psychophysical, but also taking account of the effect of drugs, of organic brain damage, and so on.

It was hypothesized that some form of "physiologic clock" (ie, a rhythmic process as interval timer) might underlie the estimation by human beings of time intervals up to about 60 seconds, and that, wherever this "clock" may be located, one might expect it to be subject to the same effects of inheritance as other biologic mechanisms. It was accordingly predicted that monozygotic (MZ)

Twin Research: Psychology and Methodology, pages 111–117

co-twins, being isogenic, would tend to have smaller intrapair psychochronometric differences than would dizygotic (DZ) co-twins.

The use of a twin-study method, despite the many criticisms leveled against such an approach, must depend in general terms on the arguments of a prosaic but compelling kind provided by Shields [1962] in defense of the field worker. Specifically, it seems reasonable to accept a substantial equivalence between twins and the general population with respect to the perception and estimation of short time intervals, since this skill, though undoubtedly affected by age, intelligence, and culture, would not be expected to be affected by any differences between the environments of twins and of singletons. It may be true that a twin method can rarely do more than show that heredity has something to do with specified individual differences, but this alone is a useful first step.

METHOD

The hypothesis was investigated using the intrapair comparison of MZ and DZ same-sex co-twins of above average intelligence, in two separate studies, using identical apparatus and procedure, but differing in the age grouping of the twins. An earlier pilot study [Grant, 1966] had shown that when prepubertal and postpubertal groups of MZ and DZ same-sex twins [5 pair MZ, 5 pair DZ, at each stage] were compared with respect to intrapair similarity on tests of short time interval estimation, there was no significant difference between the zygosities at the prepubertal stage. However, with a postpubertal group some interesting interzygosity differences were indicated.

Zygosity diagnosis in all cases was carried out by a battery of tests including a comprehensive family history, a polysymptomatic assessment, Husén's method of photography, phenylthiocarbamide tasting, and analysis of dermal ridge patterns.

Subjects

In the first study the subjects were 46 pairs of MZ and same-sex DZ co-twins, aged 14–18 years, all unmarried, living with their co-twin, and attending the same school as their co-twin. They all lay above the 75th percentile with respect to IQ. Further, as the distribution of intelligence within the total twin population is positively skewed when compared with the normal curve for the population of singletons, the experimental subjects were more highly selected with regard to the twin population than even the above percentile ranking would suggest.

In the second study the subjects were 22 pairs of MZ and same-sex DZ co-twins, aged 30–50 years, all married and living apart from their co-twin. Though not as highly selected academically as the younger group, and screened intellectually only on a short IQ test, all appeared to be of somewhat above average ability as judged by their occupational attainments.

In both studies the zygosity groups were approximately evenly divided with regard to sex. Females were not tested during menstruation.

Procedure

All experiments were carried out in a custom-built sound-proof room, with fluorescent lighting and a faint background of white noise. Wristwatches were removed before the beginning of the experimental session. While one twin was being tested, the other was involved in other activities in another room several yards away.

A number of experiments were carried out, each consisting of several series of trials, the series from one experiment being interspersed with those of others in a prearranged order. Only two experiments will be described here, involving *reproduction* [a differential sensitivity method, in which, as it does not involve conceptual mediation, error must be explained in terms of just noticeable differences (jnds) rather than the subject's time units] and *operative estimation* (a magnitude production method, a form of ratio scaling) respectively. (For details see Grant [1967a, 1967b].)

In the experiment on *reproduction,* the intervals used were 3, 5, 7, 11, 17, 28, 36, 43, 50, and 54 seconds, presented as filled auditory time, with a time pause of 3 seconds between stimulus interval and response interval. The apparatus was a transistorized impulse-producing and counting unit attached to a Venner Millisecond Stopclock (Type TSA 331-4). The subjects were simply required to switch off the buzzer after what seemed to them to be a period similar to the stimulus interval. The series were presented in random, ascending, and descending order.

In the experiment on *operative estimation* the intervals used were the same as for reproduction; the time gap ranged from 1 to 4 seconds, and the apparatus was an encased silent stopwatch, so fitted that the subject could start and stop it from the rear by means of a lever. Thus the time intervals were empty, but delimited by very brief clicks, and by movement of the fingers.

RESULTS

It will be deduced from the foregoing description that, although the raw data consisted of estimate scores, the aim in obtaining these data was to find the intrapair difference for each interval under various modal and methodologic conditions. It would be expected that most estimates would be in error, sometimes slight and sometimes very considerable. Further, this error could be either positive or negative. However, since the concern is with the distance between two scores, the calculation of the intrapair difference is simply a matter of the subtraction of the smaller score from the larger, if both have the same direction of error, or the addition of the error scores if one twin gives an underestimate and the co-twin an overestimate.

Study 1

Analysis of the data shows that with the method of reproduction, out of 30 intrapair differences, 19 are significant at the 0.05 level (Table I). Interval length does not appear to be relevant, within the narrow range studied, but there is some slight variation between methods of programming trials. It has often been claimed that, unlike methods of time estimation which depend on the use of verbalized units and which rely on a highly conceptualized type of judgment, presupposing a fairly advanced level of intellectual development, the method of reproduction "seems to provide a more direct measure of the subjective experience of time which presumably underlies the intellectualized verbal judgment" [Danziger and du Preez, 1963, p 880]. However, this assumption is questionable, and it is unwise to extrapolate from reproduction to other methods of time judgment. Further, it is well established that the method of reproduction yields low reliability from session to session.

In the case of *operative estimation* (Table II), the null hypothesis is rejected at the 0.01 level in every instance. It is noteworthy that the manner of programming trials appears to have more effect than in the case of reproduction, perhaps because the test is fairly intellectually demanding and more sensitive to small changes in set. There were no significant sex differences under either methodological condition.

In summary, there is considerable evidence in the case of the method of reproduction, and clear evidence with the method of operative estimation, that the intrapair similarity for short-interval time estimation is significantly greater for MZ co-twins than for same-sex DZ co-twins, within the age range of 14–18.

Study 2

The data for the older age group show no difference significant at the 0.05 level.

DISCUSSION

When faced with apparently paradoxical results our dilemma is initially to decide what it is that needs to be explained: The difference between Study 1 and Study 2, or some feature within one or both of the studies. Sample sizes were adequate, and the use of nonparametric statistics minimized assumptions. Study 1 subjects were traced through school records and asked to participate, and only one pair declined to do so. In Study 2 subjects were selected from a pool obtained by newspaper advertising, in terms of above-average educational and/or occupational attainments. It is difficult to conceive of any sampling bias here being

TABLE I. The Effect of Zygosity on Intrapair Differences in Estimation of Short Time Intervals Under Random, Ascending, and Descending Orders of Presentation — Method of Reproduction

Interval (seconds)	Monozygotic		Dizygotic			
	Mean intrapair differences	SD	Mean intrapair differences	SD	U	
random						
3	0.41	0.271	0.61	0.337	350	*
5	1.07	1.208	1.20	0.690	335	
7	1.22	0.539	1.56	0.847	339	*
11	2.20	1.537	2.49	1.148	304.5	
17	3.19	1.991	4.47	1.849	361.5	*
28	5.66	7.372	5.69	3.759	308.5	
36	6.26	3.966	5.53	3.800	240	
43	6.43	3.633	9.72	4.625	373.5	**
50	9.09	6.044	10.26	6.996	284	
54	7.56	5.958	12.30	6.458	380	**
ascending						
3	0.49	0.252	0.69	0.329	349	*
5	0.56	0.334	0.97	0.518	384.5	**
7	1.03	0.522	1.55	0.894	368.5	*
11	1.33	0.709	2.33	1.453	379.5	**
17	2.70	1.560	3.39	1.702	341.5	
28	4.50	2.398	5.76	3.002	331	
36	6.01	3.402	7.53	4.673	312.5	
43	6.55	2.895	8.63	4.184	349	*
50	7.70	4.999	9.89	5.524	337	
54	8.05	5.738	10.84	7.176	316.5	
descending						
3	0.51	0.392	0.64	0.449	307.5	
5	0.71	0.395	1.29	0.831	371	**
7	0.88	0.455	1.88	1.079	414.5	**
11	2.16	1.919	3.55	2.219	366.5	*
17	3.04	1.945	4.20	2.310	312	
28	4.72	2.128	7.36	4.297	360.5	*
36	5.76	2.735	8.27	4.543	353	*
43	6.23	3.637	11.56	6.788	389.5	**
50	7.57	3.813	10.67	6.388	342.5	*
54	9.56	5.663	13.88	7.152	349.5	*

*$p < 0.05$ Mann-Whitney U test.
**$p < 0.01$.

relevant to the topic under investigation. Both studies were carried out by the same investigator, and any experimenter expectancy effect would surely be almost constant, despite a six-year interval between the studies.

TABLE II. The Effect of Zygosity on Intrapair Differences in Estimation of Short Time Intervals Under Random, Ascending, and Descending Orders of Presentation — Method of Operative Estimation

| Interval (seconds) | Monozygotic | | Dizygotic | | |
	Mean intrapair differences	SD	Mean intrapair differences	SD	U
3	0.68	0.356	2.06	1.372	460	**
5	1.01	0.364	2.96	1.766	486.5	**
7	1.10	0.568	4.99	2.355	517	**
11	2.11	1.076	6.23	3.141	497	**
17	3.80	2.206	8.07	4.133	442	**
28	4.01	2.520	10.56	4.390	473.5	**
36	6.78	2.757	13.50	8.698	421	**
43	7.66	3.984	17.85	10.550	426	**
50	10.45	4.509	16.55	8.245	394	**
54	8.30	4.196	17.40	8.682	438.5	**
ascending						
3	0.62	0.535	1.21	0.661	417.5	**
5	0.93	0.449	2.53	1.186	484.5	**
7	1.19	0.583	3.52	1.564	478	**
11	2.29	0.934	5.27	2.798	449.5	**
17	3.45	1.105	7.27	4.132	407	**
28	5.15	3.719	10.90	6.166	424	**
36	8.66	5.987	17.86	9.646	419	**
43	8.56	5.441	21.42	9.977	452	**
50	9.77	4.491	22.42	13.744	410	**
54	11.66	7.696	24.51	13.552	416	**
descending						
3	0.63	0.328	2.55	1.870	466	**
5	0.82	0.416	3.84	2.310	517.5	**
7	1.25	0.919	6.09	3.536	520	**
11	1.41	1.339	7.32	4.010	481.5	**
17	3.87	2.159	10.23	6.234	477.5	**
28	3.64	2.758	15.42	9.762	488	**
36	6.28	3.736	14.85	9.199	454	**
43	7.77	5.874	19.46	10.576	462.5	**
50	9.39	11.957	21.22	10.602	467	**
54	10.85	5.376	21.51	9.896	429.5	**

**p < Mann-Whitney U test.

Zygosity diagnosis, though detailed, lacked access to medical facilities, including blood sampling, and so may have involved an occasional error, but surely not of a degree to explain such disparate results. As in most psychological experiments, a relatively limited number of measurements was taken from each subject (3 per interval, for 10 different intervals, under each of 2 experimental conditions) — yet if one attempts to obtain more, one is faced with fatigue, boredom, noncooperation, judgment drift, and so on. Thus any indication of a zygosity difference would be relatively crude, ie, any difference found is likely to be really greater than obtained data indicate.

The only consistently differentiating factors between the two studies appear to be those of subject age and of co-residence or separate residence. Developmental research on time estimation has consistently shown that children only gradually achieve the capacity to estimate duration reasonably accurately, dependent on both maturational and cognitive factors. An adult level of skill is usually attained by the early teens. While temporal values may change with increasing age, there has been no evidence of changes in accuracy of time estimation except in cases of physiologic disorder or brain damage. However, this assumption of stability may be misleading because it is based on group averages rather than on longitudinal studies of individuals.

Differentiation by age may be expected to increase intrapair dissimilarity, but the crucial factor may be that of co-residence or separate residence. We are only gradually beginning to understand the effect of physiologic and behavioral rhythms, but we know the problems which can arise when a day-active person is married to a night-active partner, or the influence of work rhythms in the employment context. MZ co-resident adolescents are likely to be more similar in both physiologic and activity patterns (presumably underlying the capacity to estimate time) than other human beings, but separation and aging will both add to dissimilarity.

The high level of MZ similarity for operative estimation in the younger age group may be partly artifactual because of the intellectually select nature of the subjects. On the other hand, a less selected group would probably have shown a greater variability and thus masked a real difference.

Clearly the case is not closed, but a definite answer appears to await detailed longitudinal studies, even if only of a few twin pairs.

REFERENCES

Cohen J (1967): "Psychological Time in Health and Disease." Springfield, Illinois: CC Thomas.

Danziger K, du Preez PD (1963): Reliability of time estimation by the method of reproduction. Percept Mot Skills 16:879–884.

Gooddy W (1959): Time and the nervous system. Lancet 2:1155–1156.

Grant E (1966): "An Experimental Study of the Possible Role of Heredity in the Estimation of Time." Doctoral thesis, University of Leicester.

Grant E (1967a): Problems of methodology in time estimation studies. Alberta Psychologist 8(1):12–25.

Grant E (1967b): Problems of terminology and psychophysics in time estimation studies. Alberta Psychologist 8(3):18–37.

Shields J (1962): Monozygotic Twins Brought Up Apart and Brought Up Together." London: Oxford University Press.

A Danish Twin Study of Manic-Depressive Disorders

A Bertelsen

INTRODUCTION

To date eight studies of twin series with manic-depressive disorders have been reported. The concordance rates (by pairs) for monozygotic twins have consistently tended to be higher than rates for dizygotic pairs, indicating a genetic factor, but the existence of a number of discordant monozygotic pairs shows that the environment also plays an important role. The rates cannot, however, be compared directly, at least not without strong reservations, because the studies are based on different methods of sampling and investigation and on varying diagnostic concepts. Furthermore, some of the studies include only small numbers of pairs. The earlier studies do not all meet the standards required for an ideally unselected and representative sample. These studies show the highest concordance rates for monozygotic pairs, which usually is explained as the result of selection among more ill twins from hospital populations with a higher chance for concordant pairs to be reported. More recent studies have found lower monozygotic concordance rates among fairly unselected and representative samples, but they include only a few pairs and are based on rather strict concepts of manic-depressive disorders. The existence of a nationwide twin register and a national psychiatric register in a small country where it is feasible to do a catamnestic study induced us to make another investigation of a series of twins with manic-depressive disorders.

MATERIALS AND METHODS

The Danish Twin Register was established by Bent Harvald and Mogens Hauge in the years 1954—1967. The twin register comprises all same-sex twin

Twin Research: Psychology and Methodology, pages 119—124

pairs born in the years 1870–1920. As far as possible the twins were traced to their present residence or to their death. All pairs of twins in which one or both of the partners had died before the age of 6 years were excluded, leaving about one-third of the twin population for investigation. A questionnaire was sent out to each of the traced twins or in case of death to the nearest living relative. The questionnaire asked about hospital admissions and various diseases and disorders including nervous and mental disorders. Answers have been obtained in nearly all cases, if necessary by supplementary personal interviews. In this way a subregister was established of twins who had been admitted to hospitals for mental disorders: The Psychiatric Twin Register.

The National Psychiatric Register was initiated in the 1920s. Through the following decades it developed into a fairly complete registration of admissions to Danish mental hospitals and psychiatric departments. In 1967 the Psychiatric Twin Register was completed by cross-matching of the Danish Twin Register with the National Psychiatric Register, which led to a supplementary inclusion of pairs with at least one member appearing in both registers. For the dead twins, death certificates have been reviewed, and cases of suicide without psychiatric classification have also been collected. The present composition of the Psychiatric Twin Register is the result of a thorough revision of all available case material.

The probands were ascertained in accordance with Kraepelin's concept of manic-depressive disorders (this rather wide concept was chosen to permit investigation of a broad variety of manic-depressive disorders). This means that those ascertained as probands are twins who have been admitted to psychiatric hospitals because of disorders that involve predominating mood disturbances of a universal character not restricted to the sphere of recent psychic traumas, and are characterized by disturbances of psychomotor and mental activity, typical characteristic sleep disturbances, and diurnal variations, and furthermore, by a periodic course and a tendency to recovery without defect. (The same criteria have, of course, been applied in the evaluation of the co-twins.)

A total of 126 probands from 110 pairs were selected in this way. To meet the standards of more narrow concepts of manic-depressive disorders, the probands have been divided into subgroups of probands with typical, atypical, and probable manic-depressive disorders. The typical manic-depressive disorders were rather strictly delineated as disorders with characteristic manic or melancholic symptoms, possibly accompanied by perplexity, delusions, disorders of perception and behavior, but all consistent with the prevailing mood. The atypical probands differed in one of two ways: The N-atypical probands displayed pronounced neurotic symptoms, such as asthenic, anxious, anancastic, or hysterical traits in cases which otherwise showed typical symptoms and course so that the diagnosis of manic-depressive disorder was certain. The S-atypical probands showed pronounced schizophrenia-like symptoms, such as delusions or disorders of perception and behavior not consistent with the prevailing mood, but still showed enough typical symptoms and course as to permit the certain diagnosis of a manic-depressive disorder. The group of probable manic-depressive disorders was more broadly defined and included disorders with sufficient typical symptoms or course to make the diagnosis of manic-depressive disorder probable but not certain: Alternative diagnoses might be reactive psychosis or neurotic disorder, but in no case would schizophrenia be suspected.

The catamnestic investigation was carried out by personal interviews of the twins or, in case of death, their nearest living relative. Of the 220 twin partners 138 were alive. They were all visited and only five refused to be interviewed. In these cases, and for the dead twins, it was possible in the main to get information from relatives or from general practitioners. Only for seven twins from four pairs who died many years ago it was not possible to get any further catamnestic information. All the interviews were performed by the same investigator. The interview was made open and without fixed structure in order to put the interviewed person at ease so that he might talk freely and spontaneously about himself. At the same time the interviewer made sure that certain relevant points were covered.

The zygosity was determined by serologic investigation in nearly all cases where both twin partners in a pair were alive. The serologic determination was based upon 16–25 independent systems of erythrocyte types, tissue types, serum protein variants, and isoenzymes. The probability of monozygosity is 0.98 or more in pairs where the partners show complete accordance. For the remaining pairs the zygosity was assessed anthropometrically from information based on questions about pronounced similarity of general appearance and about mistaken identities by others. The reliability of this method has been estimated by Hauge et al [1968] to be above 0.95 for monozygosity in cases of consistently positive answers to both questions and for dizygosity in cases where the answers are consistently negative, or one answer negative and the other doubtful. In all other cases zygosity was considered as undetermined.

RESULTS

Of the 110 pairs, 55 were found to be monozygotic and 52 to be dizygotic. For three pairs the information was insufficient to determine the zygosity and these pairs have been discarded from the concordance analysis. The 55 monozygotic pairs included 14 in which both twins were probands. The 52 dizygotic pairs included two pairs in which both twins were probands.

The concordance has been evaluated at two levels, the strict concordance or C_1, and the broad concordance or C_2. In the strict concordance the co-twin has a diagnosis of manic-depressive disorder, certain or probable, irrespective of polarity or severity. The broad concordance includes co-twins with the diagnoses of psychosis other than manic-depressive disorder, of pronounced affective personality disorder, and of suicide. The concordance has been calculated as the proband rate and as the direct pairwise rate. (The proband concordance is the proportion of probands with affected co-twins.) Among the co-twins of 69 monozygotic probands were found 46 with manic-depressive disorders, resulting in a monozygotic proband rate of 0.67. Among the co-twins of 54 dizygotic probands, 11 had manic-depressive disorders, which gives a dizygotic proband rate of 0.20. The corresponding proband rates of broad (C_2) concordance were for the monozygotic twins 0.87 and for the dizygotic twins 0.37. (The proband concordance rate is the more appropriate measure of concordance in studies based on independently ascertained index cases representative of a defined population and it yields figures comparable with risk figures of relatives and of the general population. The direct concordance rate by pairs is the proportion of pairs with both twins affected.) Among 55 monozygotic pairs 32 were found concordant as to manic-depressive disorder, yielding a monozygotic rate by pairs of 0.58. Among 52 dizygotic pairs, 9 pairs were found concordant, resulting in a dizygotic pairwise rate of 0.17. The corresponding rates of broad (C_2) concordance were 0.82 for monozygotic pairs and 0.33 for dizygotic pairs. When only hospitalized cases among the co-twins are taken into consideration in the evaluation of concordance, the proband rate of strict concordance is 0.52 for monozygotic twins and 0.13 for dizygotic twins, and the broad concordance rates are 0.65 and 0.26, respectively. The differences between the rates by pairs are all highly significant and support the previous findings of a strong genetic factor. Age correction is not shown but has been calculated by the Slater method for twin pairs. It resulted in only small increases of 1 or 2 in the last digits, because of the age of the sample and the length of observation.

The number of years between the onset of illness in the proband and in the co-twin varied widely, by as much as 30–45 years. But more than half of the concordant monozygotic co-twins had become ill within 8 years and there was a significantly positive correlation between the ages of onset in the concordant monozygotic twins.

With respect to sex the concordance rates were quite similar. The concordance rates for probands with typical, atypical, and probable manic-depressive disorder show remarkable trends. For the typical probands the rates are about the same as the rates of the total sample. For the atypical probands the monozygotic rate is somewhat higher. This holds true for the N-atypical as well as for the S-atypical probands, perhaps because of an additional effect of a co-existing disorder of environmental or of genetic origin. The probable group shows somewhat lower rates as well for the monozygotic as for the dizygotic twins. This could be explained by a possible inclusion of cases with reactive depression or elation disguised as endogenous depression or manic psychosis. An alternative explanation is a polygenic heredity with a lower genetic loading for this group, demanding precipitating traumas for the manifestation of the disorder.

The proband concordance has also been calculated with respect to bipolar and unipolar forms of disorder. Bipolar disorders were defined as disorders with at least one episode of elated mood including hypomania with the exception of short and transient episodes following electroshock treatment. A case of pure mania was thus included in this group. Unipolar disorders were defined as disorders with episodes of depression only, irrespective of the degree of depression or the number of episodes. The monozygotic proband rates clearly tend to be lower for the unipolar probands than for the bipolar probands on both levels of concordance, whereas the dizygotic rates are about the same. When the probands were further divided into probands with mania and probands with hypomania, and into probands with three or more episodes of depression and probands with less than three episodes of depression, the rates showed some remarkable differences. First, the monozygotic rates were found to be almost identical for probands with mania and hypomania, which supports the assumption that hypomania is as good an indicator of bipolar disorder as clearly manic symptoms. Second, probands with fewer than three episodes of depression showed lower rates than probands with three or more episodes of depression, who have rates of nearly the same size as the total sample. This finding supports a sharper definition of unipolar disease, demanding at least three separate episodes of depression in accordance with the definition of Perris [1966].

The distribution of the monozygotic concordant pairs with respect to polarity shows a high number of pairs in which both partners are either unipolar or bipolar concordant — 11 and 14, respectively. Only seven concordant pairs have one twin unipolar and the other bipolar. This distribution is quite remarkable. If we assume that unipolar and bipolar forms are genetically completely identical, the expected binomial distribution, based upon the observed ratio of unipolar to bipolar cases, will result in significantly different figures. The unipolar and bipolar forms then cannot be completely indistinguishable in genetic respects. There seems to be some kind of heterogeneity, but whether the difference is due to specific or modifying genes cannot be evaluated from monozygotic twin pairs. Only dizygotic twin pairs or family studies will allow an evaluation of this problem. The dizygotic pairs in the present study have too small numbers of concordant pairs to show any significant trends, and their distribution as to polarity gives no support to the hypothesis of two genetically separate diseases. The 11 unipolar concordant monozygotic pairs are all females. Recent family studies have also found a preponderance of unipolar females, suggesting a sex dependence of the unipolar disorder. In 9 of the 11 concordant female pairs of the present sample, the depressive episodes were related to pregnancy and childbirth or the climacteric, which are specifically female experiences that suggest an endocrine factor.

SUMMARY

A catamnestic investigation of an unselected and representative sample of twins with manic-depressive disorders has resulted in a monozygotic proband concordance of 0.67 and a pairwise concordance of 0.58, and a dizygotic proband concordance of 0.20 and a pairwise concordance of 0.18. The difference between the monozygotic and dizygotic pairs is significant at the 0.001 level, which confirms the evidence of a strong genetic factor.

An analysis of the distribution of the concordant monozygotic pairs with respect to unipolar and bipolar forms yields figures far from those expected for completely identical genetics and thus suggests some kind of heterogeneity.

REFERENCES

Bertelsen A, Harvald B, Hauge M (1977): A Danish twin study of manic-depressive disorders. Br J Psychiatry 130:330–351.

Hauge et al (1968): The Danish Twin Registry. Acta Genet Med Gemellol (Roma) 17:315–332.

Perris C (1966): A study of bipolar (manic-depressive) and unipolar recurrent depressive psychoses. Acta Psychiatr Scand (Suppl 194).

Contribution of Twin Studies to Psychiatric Nosology

Svenn Torgersen

INTRODUCTION

In psychiatric twin research, the classical twin method has been used extensively. The main aim of these studies is to elucidate the relative importance of environmental and hereditary factors in the development of psychiatric states. The method takes advantage of the biological fact that there are two types of twins; dizygotic (DZ) with more or less dissimilar genetic makeup, and monozygotic (MZ) with identical genetic endowment. In addition, it is assumed that the similarity in environment is more or less the same in MZ and DZ twin pairs.

From this kind of research another development has emerged. In genetic thinking it is common to operate with the concepts of "genotype" and "phenotype." The phenotype can vary even if the genotype is the same. Identification of the spectrum of phenotypes possible in the same genotype may be of considerable significance, since it might be the starting point for preventive work as well as a clue to a more logical nosologic system founded on etiology.

In the following, I shall give some examples from psychiatric research and argue that the rationale of this type of research does not depend on whether the basic assumptions of the classical twin method are true or not. Finally I shall present some data from my own research.

Ever since Leonhard [1959] proposed to separate endogenous depressions into bipolar (manic-depressive) and unipolar (depressive) types the question of how fruitful this separation is has been a subject of debate.

Endogenous Depression

If unipolar and bipolar depressions were possible phenotypes stemming from the same genotype, one would expect that the co-twin of an MZ proband with a unipolar depression could develop bipolar as well as unipolar depression. In DZ

Twin Research: Psychology and Methodology, pages 125–130

pairs one would expect the same, although the concordance would be smaller for all three combinations of depressions (unipolar-unipolar, bipolar-bipolar, and unipolar-bipolar).

If unipolar and bipolar depressions are phenotypes of different genotypes, one would expect few, if any, MZ pairs where one twin partner displayed a unipolar and the other a bipolar depression. In DZ twin pairs, on the other hand, one would find relatively more combinations of unipolar-bipolar depressions in co-twins.

In their extensive twin study of endogenous depressions Bertelsen, Harvald, and Hauge [1977] found in fact that in MZ pairs both twins mostly developed the same depressive state. More rarely did one observe pairs where one twin had a unipolar and the co-twin had a bipolar depression. In DZ twin pairs, on the other hand, the combination of unipolar-bipolar depressions was found just as frequently as unipolar-unipolar, and bipolar-bipolar combinations. The results of the Bertelsen study were in accordance with earlier studies of far smaller twin samples.

The conclusion seems natural that unipolar and bipolar depression are related to different genotypes and accordingly ought to be separated nosologically, as Leonhard proposed.

Schizophrenia

It has been maintained — perhaps most clearly articulated by Meehl [1962] — that schizophrenia and the nonschizophrenic schizoid personality type are closely related, clinical schizophrenia being a more serious phenotype of the schizoid genotype. If this were the case, one would expect a preponderance of schizoid personalities in co-twins of MZ schizophrenics and a somewhat lower incidence in the co-twins of DZ schizophrenics.

The results of different studies are somewhat conflicting. However, studies where schizoid personality traits are evaluated more systematically and objectively find slight support for such a hypothesis [Mosher, Stabenau, and Pollin, 1971; Gottesman and Shields, 1972]. Accordingly, there is no clear evidence that schizophrenia and schizoid personality are related nosologically.

A Reformulation of the Basic Assumption

In the studies reported, the basic assumption has been the same as in the classic twin method: While MZ twin partners are identical in genetic equipment, the similarity in environment of MZ twin partners is basically the same as for DZ twin partners. However, this assumption has been seriously challenged. MZ twin partners spend more time together, they are more stongly identified with each other, they are more similar in physique and appearance, and hence they receive more similar reactions from the environment.

The conclusion might be that the use of the twin samples in nosologic research is questionable. I shall argue that this is not necessarily so.

Whether one considers the higher concordance in MZ twin partners to be a result of identical genetic equipment, or whether one ascribes a differential concordance to highly similar environment in childhood and later, or both, it is to be agreed that MZ twin partners are influenced by more similar etiologic factors than DZ twin partners in their developmental history. Hence, even if the basic assumption of the classical twin method is questionable, an analysis of concordance and discordance in twin pairs may give a clue to an etiologically based nosology. Two different psychiatric states met more frequently in the two partners of MZ twin pairs compared to DZ twin pairs ought to have similar etiology and hence should be nosologically related. Conversely, two psychiatric states met more seldom in the partners of concordant MZ pairs, and more frequently in the partners of concordant DZ pairs, probably have a different etiology and should be separated nosologically. It is still not claimed that hereditary factors are important in the etiology. It can be subtle environmental factors affecting MZ, but not DZ twin partners, in the same way because of the close relationship of MZ partners in childhood.

THE PRESENT STUDY

Sample and Method

Presently I am carrying out a large-scale study of neurotic twins in Norway. The sample has been obtained by checking patient registers of inpatient and outpatient psychiatric clinics all over the country with the National Twin Registry.* Up to now, 212 MZ and DZ female and male twin pairs have been personally interviewed. In assessing the psychiatric state of the subject the so-called Present State Examination (PSE) has been employed [Wing, Cooper, and Sartorius 1974]. The diagnoses are, however, not yet arrived at by means of computer, and for the time being they represent my own global evaluation. The final zygosity diagnosis will be determined by means of blood and serum typing. However, the preliminary results are based on a mailed questionnaire. The correlation between questionnaires and serologic testing is high, however, so it is not to be expected that the final zygosity diagnosis will be much different from what is assumed in this paper [Cederlöf, 1966]. Still, the report must be considered as preliminary.

The Research Question

In the psychiatric literature it has been debated whether it is worthwhile to distinguish neurotic depression from anxiety neurosis [Derogatis, Klerman, and Lipman, 1972].

---

*Dr. Einar Kringlen is in charge of the registry of twins born before January 1, 1946, and Dr. Kåre Berg is in charge of register of twins born in subsequent years.

If one could demonstrate that these neurotic conditions had different etiologies, one could argue for a nosologic differentiation. According to the logic presented previously, this would be the case if one found that both twins mostly showed a neurotic depression or that both twins displayed anxiety neurosis in concordant MZ twin pairs. In relatively few MZ twin pairs would one twin have a neurotic depression and the co-twin an anxiety state. In DZ pairs, on the other hand, one would expect relatively more twin pairs of which one twin showed a neurotic depression and the other one had an anxiety neurosis.

RESULTS AND DISCUSSION

In calculating the concordance rate I have used the probandwise method, because it is the more appropriate measure of concordance in studies based on independently ascertained index cases, representative of a defined population [Allen, Harvald, and Shields, 1967].

Table I shows that the co-twin of MZ probands with a neurotic depression often also develops a neurotic depression. Correspondingly, the co-twin of the proband with anxiety neurosis also shows a picture of anxiety neurosis. The problem however, is, that quite a few pairs exhibit a neurotic depression in one twin and anxiety neurosis in the co-twin. Turning to the dizygotic group one finds much the same picture, apart from fewer pairs in which both display anxiety neurosis. The result in Table I does not clearly speak for a difference in etiology between depressive and anxiety neurosis.

In Table II, I have restricted the analysis to pairs in which the probands show chronic depression or chronic anxiety. Probands with milder reactive depressions and anxiety states of shorter duration have been excluded. Now one can observe a more clear distinction between MZ and DZ twin pairs. In MZ twin pairs there are no co-twins of chronic depressives who display an anxiety state of any kind. Con-

TABLE I. Relationship Between Diagnoses of Anxiety and Depression in Probands and Diagnoses in Co-twins

Diagnoses of probands		Diagnoses of co-twins				
		Depression	Anxiety	Other psychiatric states	Normal	N
MZ	Depression	12 (27.3)	5 (11.4)	2 (4.5)	25 (56.8)	44 (100.0)
	Anxiety	3 (10.0)	9 (30.0)	2 (6.7)	16 (53.3)	30 (100.0)
DZ	Depression	18 (31.0)	3 (5.2)	6 (10.3)	31 (53.5)	58 (100.0)
	Anxiety	7 (12.5)	5 (8.9)	4 (7.1)	40 (71.4)	56 (99.9)

TABLE II. Relationship Between Diagnoses of Chronic Depression and Chronic Anxiety in Probands and Diagnoses in Co-Twins

Diagnoses of probands		Diagnoses of co-twins				
		Depression	Anxiety	Other psychiatric states	Normal	N
MZ	Chronic depression	4 (36.4)	0	1 (9.1)	6 (54.5)	11 (100.0)
MZ	Chronic anxiety	1 (8.3)	7 (58.3)	2 (16.7)	2 (16.7)	12 (100.0)
DZ	Chronic depression	1 (25.8)	2 (6.5)	5 (16.1)	16 (51.6)	31 (100.0)
	Chronic anxiety	3 (13.0)	2 (8.7)	0	18 (78.3)	23 (100.0)

versely, in MZ probands with chronic anxiety neurosis, one comes across only one co-twin showing a depressive neurosis.

In contrast, in DZ twin pairs one finds two probands with chronic depression, whose co-twin has an anxiety neurosis, and three probands with a chronic anxiety neurosis whose co-twin has a neurotic depression. The explanation is that MZ probands with milder reactive neurotic depression or MZ probands with milder reactive anxiety neurosis had co-twins with different affective reactions.

CONCLUSIONS

Even if the numbers are small, it is perhaps warranted to suggest that the etiology of chronic neurotic depression is different from the etiology of anxiety states. Furthermore, the etiology of chronic anxiety neurosis is different from the etiology of neurotic depressive states. However, in milder reactive affective states, it is not possible to differentiate anxiety and depressive states etiologically.

Hence, it may be fruitful to separate chronic neurotic depression and chronic anxiety neurosis nosologically. Milder reactive neurotic depression and anxiety states, however, might preferably be considered to be in an intermediate position between these two affective poles (Fig 1).

To return to the main point, nothing has been said about the nature of the etiologic difference between the two chronic affective states. It may be heredity or subtile environmental factors affecting MZ twin partners uniformly in early childhood or later.

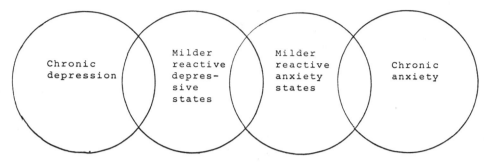

Fig. 1. A model of a nosologic differentiation of affective neurotic states.

REFERENCES

Allen G, Harvald B, Shields J (1967): Measures of twin concordance. Acta Genet Stat Med 17:475–481.

Bertelsen A, Harvald B, Hauge M (1977): A Danish twin study of manic-depressive disorders. Br J Psychiatr 130:330–351.

Cederlöf R (1966): "The Twin Method in Epidemiological Studies of Chronic Disease." Stockholm: Institute of Hygiene of the Karolinska Institute.

Derogatis LR, Kierman GL, Lipman RS (1972): Anxiety states and depressive neuroses. Issues in nosological discrimination. J Nerv Ment Dis 155:392–403.

Gottesman II, Shields J (1972): "Schizophrenia and Genetics. A Twin Study Vantage Point." New York: Academic.

Leonard K (1959): "Aufteilung der endogenen Psychosen." Berlin: Akademie-Verlag.

Meehl PE (1962): Schizotaxia, schizotypy and schizophrenia. Am Psychol 17:827–838.

Mosher LR, Stabenau JR, Pollin W (1971): "Schizoidness in the Nonschizophrenics." Paper presented at the Fifth World Congress of Psychiatry, Mexico City, December 1971.

Wing JK, Cooper JE, Sartorius N (1974): "Measurement and Classification of Psychiatric symptoms." London: Cambridge University Press.

A Behavioral Study of Twins With Coronary Heart Disease

Einar Kringlen

INTRODUCTION

Coronary heart disease (CHD) represents one of the great medical challenges today on a level with cancer and mental disorders. The increase in the incidence of coronary heart disease over the last 50 years in most Western countries and the great variation in frequency in different regions of the world speak for the significance of environmental factors in the etiology. Any alteration of the gene pool in such a short period of time is out of the question. Furthermore, twin studies support this view, since the difference in concordance rates in monozygotic (MZ) and dizygotic (DZ) twins with regard to coronary heart disease is negligible. Harvald and Hauge [1965] observed higher concordance rates in MZ than in DZ twins with respect to deaths caused by myocardial infarction. However, the difference was slight and statistically not significant for male pairs.

No specific environmental factors of etiologic significance have been identified. Epidemiologic research has, true enough, discovered a series of "risk factors" in CHD. Risk, however, is not the same as cause. Research has shown that factors such as age, blood pressure, cholesterol, cigarette smoking, body weight, exercise are correlated with development of CHD. However only age, systolic blood pressure, and cholesterol are universally accepted as risk factors.

In this situation a study of twins discordantly affected with CHD might help solve the problem of etiology by asking which factors discriminate between twin partners in discordant pairs. Twins have not only the same age and basically the same family milieu but in case of MZ twins also the same genes, including the same sex. By comparing twins of which one is a smoker, and the other a nonsmoker, it is possible to investigate the etiologic significance of smoking. By

Twin Research: Psychology and Methodology, pages 131–135

comparing twins where one partner is hard-working, whereas the other is more relaxed, one can examine the influence of work behavior on the development of coronary heart diseases.

Cederlöf, Jonsson, and Kaij [1966] investigated the influence of smoking on bronchitis and angina pectoris. First twins as single individuals were considered and a positive correlation between smoking and bronchitis and between smoking and angina pectoris was noted. However, by comparing twins belonging to the same pair, but with dissimilar smoking habits, they were able to confirm the etiologic significance of smoking on respiratory symptoms, but not on angina pectoris.

These findings are supported by a clinical study of 200 twin pairs discordant for smoking carried out by Lundman [1966]. According to this author cigarette smoking per se most likely had no etiologic relationship to coronary heart disease, nor did he find that smoking caused hypertension, elevated blood cholesterol or triglyceride.

In another Swedish study, by Liljefors [1970], 91 male twin pairs (51 MZ and 40 DZ), aged 42–67, were located of which one or both twins had symptoms of coronary heart disease. This author could observe no relationship between cigarette smoking and symptoms of coronary insufficiency. A slight negative correlation could be observed with regard to physical exercise and coronary symptoms. It was discovered, however, that in pairs discordant for coronary symptoms the ill twin had experienced more financial problems. Furthermore, strong ambition and overtime work were more frequently observed in twins with coronary infarction than in well partners. In fact, it was an outstanding finding that the more seriously affected twin in MZ pairs had been the more dedicated to work.

PRESENT STUDY

Sample

Names of approximately 10,000 patients aged 40–69 years admitted to medical wards of the larger general hospitals in Norway with coronary heart disease (myocardial infarction and angina pectoris) during the period 1971–75 were checked against our national twin register (Kringlen, 1978). After exclusion of pairs one of whom had died before the age of 40, a sample of 78 MZ and DZ pairs of twins remained.

METHODS

After identification of the index-twin a letter was mailed to the twin through the hospital where the patient had been treated. The twin was asked to participate in the study and requested to fill out a short questionnaire regarding zygosity and name and address of co-twin. The next step was to carry out a personal interview of the twins. Since the twins were living at various places around the country, this involved a lot of work. At the present time, half of the twins have been investigated. The interview is semistructured and lasts approximately one hour, covering life history with particular emphasis on work habits, life style, and personality problems. In addition blood pressure is measured in sitting position during the end of the visit. A venous blood sample is also taken for determination of cholesterol and zygosity diagnosis. In case of death, information is sought from the family and the remaining twin. In addition information is supplemented by medical records from physicians and hospitals.

PRELIMINARY RESULTS

Since only part of the twins have been interviewed, I shall limit myself to a presentation of some preliminary impressions.

First of all I was struck, as a psychiatrist, by the "normality" of the subjects. Few twins have manifested clear-cut neurotic or psychotic symptoms or drinking behavior. As a group these subjects present a picture of conscientious, hard-working people – pillars of society.

The numbers are small and the difference is not statistically significant, but in both MZ and DZ discordantly affected pairs the twin with coronary heart disease has smoked more, worked harder, and experienced more personal problems related to work or family than his co-twin.

In the following I shall give a summary of the life history of two MZ pairs, discordant for coronary heart disease.

Male MZ Pair, Born 1910

Twin A suffers from coronary heart disease; twin B; no coronary symptoms. The twins are Nos. 4 and 5 of eleven children. They grew up partly on a farm and partly in a small village where their father was running a small factory.

Twin A married at 26 years of age a widow ten years older than himself, whereas twin B went to sea. From the age of 15 twin A worked as a salesman and since the age of 26 he has run his own business. After some years as a seaman, twin B has been a construction worker.

Both twins have been hard-working people. However, twin A has experienced considerably more stress in his work than twin B. For many years A commuted long distances between two towns, which in practice meant that in some periods he worked both day and night. Twin B has always had regular work hours.

Twin A married at 26 years of age a widow ten years older than himself. The couple has no children. The relationship has been relatively satisfactory, except for a period ten years ago, when they were separated for three years.

Twin B married at the age of 42 and has obviously experienced his martial relationship as satisfactory.

Both twins are by nature kind and extroverted and both are persons of orderly, regular habits. Both twins are active and somewhat restless — perhaps twin B is more so. Both are easily moved by sad events. Twin A, for instance, never attends a funeral. Twin A drinks more than twin B, but none of them has directly misused alcohol.

Neither of the twins has experienced extreme hardships in life, except for A, who 20 years ago suffered a financial crisis with ensuing personal problems for two to three years. Neither of the twins has suffered serious psychiatric symptoms.

Today both have moderate hypertension — A 180/120, and B 200/110. Both have elevated blood cholesterol — A 8.4 and B 9.7 mmoles/liter. Both have been smoking for 50 years — A approximately 15 cigarettes per day, B six cigarettes a day. Twin B has had more exercise in his free time than A.

Twin A developed an acute myocardial infarction for the first time in 1974 at the age of 64. Two years later he suffered two more attacks, and since then he has been troubled by angina pectoris during exercise and emotional excitement.

Comment. A male MZ pair, aged 67, discordant for coronary heart disease has been described. The most noteworthy difference in the twins' life histories is related to work. Twin A has lived a considerably more restless and stressful life than his twin brother, with irregular rhythm and long working hours. With regard to cholesterol, blood pressure, smoking, and exercise the differences are slight.

Female MZ Pair, Born 1905

Twin A has coronary symptoms; twin B is symptom-free. The twins are Nos. 8 and 9 of nine children. They grew up under rather poor conditions on a small farm in western Norway. As a child twin A was the dominant and the more independent of the twins — a role relationship which has continued into adulthood. She moved in with an elder sister to help with her children at the age of 10, whereas twin B stayed at home with her parents till she had finished school at 14 years of age. Neither of the twins received any formal education after elementary school.

Twin A developed a peptic ulcer at the age of 17—18 after a period of hard work. At the age of 23 she married a small-property owner and had four children. Her husband died in 1952 of cancer.

Twin A seems to have been an extroverted and independent woman with social interests and has never experienced manifest mental problems. She has always worked hard, in particular after she lost her husband, when she had to take total responsibility for family and farm. Often she had to work from early morning till midnight.

At the age of 62 twin A had her first attack of myocardial infarction. The next attack came in 1970. Since 1973 she has been suffereing from angina pectoris. However, the last two years she has been without symptoms.

Twin B married when 21 years old. Her husband worked both as fisherman and as a rod worker. The couple did not have any children and twin B had, compared with her twin sister, a rather quiet and protected life without much work.

Compared with her sister twin B has been more reserved and more dependent, more restless and more emotionally labile. She developed moderate hypertension at the age of 62, but her blood pressure normalized rapidly after drug therapy. At times during the last nine years she has felt difficulty in breathing and slight chest pains, symptoms which obviously have a psychologic origin, probably caused by worrying and identification with her twin sister.

Neither of the twins is a smoker. Both have slight hypertension today — twin A 170/120 and twin B 150/100. Both have mildly elevated cholesterol levels — twin A 8.7 and twin B 6.8 mmoles/liter.

Comment. Twin A, who developed coronary heart disease, has higher blood pressure and higher blood cholesterol than twin B. However, the difference is negligible. The most remarkable dissimilarity in this pair seems to be related, as in the former case, to stress and work habits. Twin A has been exposed to considerably more psychic strain and drudgery than her twin sister. She has been obliged to work hard all her life, and at the age of 47 she lost her husband.

REFERENCES

Cederlöf R, Jonsson E, Kaij L (1966): Respiratory symptoms and "angina pectoris" in twins with reference to smoking habits: An epidemiological study with mailed questionnaires. Arch Environ Health 13:743.

Harvald B, Hauge M (1965): Hereditary factors elucidated by twin studies. In Neel JV, Shaw MW, Schull WJ (eds): "Genetics and the Epidemiology of Chronic Diseases." Washington DC: US Department of Health, Education, and Welfare.

Kringlen E (1978): Norwegian Twin Registers. These procedings, Part B, "Biology and Epidemiology."

Liljefors I (1970): Coronary heart disease in male twins. Hereditary and environmental factors in concordant and discordant pairs. Acta Med Scand (Supplement 511).

Lundman T (1966): Smoking in relation to coronary heart disease and lung function in twins. A co-twin control study. Acta Med Scand 180 (Supplement 455).

Intrapair Variations in Intelligence Test Scores Among Mentally Retarded Monozygotic and Dizygotic Twin Pairs Reared Apart

Diane Sank, with the assistance of Brian D Sank Firschein

Mentally retarded twins provide a useful method for analyzing the etiology of intellectual retardation in humans. Mentally retarded (MR) twins also may permit a different perspective on the question of the range of potential and/or actual intelligence (ie, IQ) as measured by the standard intelligence tests used in the United States.

We have attempted to explore this range of human intelligence, as reflected by IQ, using a population of mentally retarded monozygotic (MZ) and dizygotic (DZ) twins from New York State, of whom all the MR index cases lived in a public institution or school for the MR. The raw data were obtained from a previous study of the etiology of mental retardation, which was completed and published by Gordon Allen with the collaboration of Franz J. Kallmann, George S. Baroff, and myself [1962] at the New York State Psychiatric Institute. Zygosity had been determined by blood groups, fingerprints, similarity data, and, in one pair, skin grafts. The present study utilized the intelligence test scores for 143 pairs of twins, consisting of 57 MZ and 86 DZ twins, in which one or both members of each pair were diagnosed as MR (having an IQ score of 69 or less). We omitted MR twins with Down syndrome, as it is a proven genetic trait attributable to a trisomy 21 or tanslocation 21 chromosome. There were 22 (15%) blacks and Puerto Ricans in this MR population. In 17 (12%) of these twin pairs the MR or normal (N) co-twin had a diagnosis of mental illness.

Intrapair (within pair) IQ point differences (IPD) were computed for each twin pair. The intrapair intelligence test scores for the 143 twin pairs were based on the most recent and chronologically closest IQ tests for each twin pair. Most of

Twin Research: Psychology and Methodology, pages 137–143

the twins were tested with the revised Stanford-Binet Intelligence Scale (S-B). The Wechsler-Bellevue (W-B) and Wechsler Intelligence Scale for Children (WISC) were also used.

Table I shows the range of actual IPD for MZ and DZ twins broken down into male (♂♂), female (♀♀), concordant (CC), and discordant (DC) for mental retardation. Also shown are the mean IQ IPD for each type of MZ and DZ twins. Of interest are the first and third rows of figures, showing MZ males (♂♂) and females (♀♀) CC for mental retardation. There are mean IPDs of 6.3 for the MZ males and 5.3 for MZ females, while IPD ranges are 0–39 IQ points for the males and 0–21 for the females.

The DZ males concordant for mental retardation (row 5) have a range and mean IPD that are comparable to those of the male MZ twins concordant for mental retardation. In contrast, the female DZ twins concordant for mental retardation (row 7) have a much larger range and mean IPD than both the female MZ twins concordant for mental retardation. The unlike-sexed DZ twins concordant for mental retardation (row 9) show an even larger range and mean IPD.

The IPD of MZ and DZ, both males and females, discordant for mental retardation probably result from 1) MR in the index case (IC), with normal IQ in the co-twin or 2) greatly different environments of the MR index case and normal co-twin (ie, institutional "home" vs natural or biological family).

Twins who are discordant for mental retardation may be considered as "mimicking" separated twins with normal IQ (ie, non-MR), as each pair consists of one normal member who is living at home, while the MR member has resided for most of his or her life in a public institution called a "state school." The latter is basically a custodial institution, belying the word "School" in its title.

TABLE I. IQ Intrapair Difference (IPD) Scores in Twins Concordant (CC) and Discordant (DC) for Mental Retardation

Mentally retarded twins	Number of pairs	Range of IPD in IQ (points)	Mean IQ IPD (points)
MZ ♂♂ CC	30	0–39	6.3
MZ ♂♂ DZ	8	45–90	64.5
MZ ♀♀ CC	15	0–21	5.3
MZ ♀♀ DC	4	63–87	73.0
DZ ♂♂ CC	15	0–31	8.5
DZ ♂♂ DC	5	29–90	63.8
DZ ♀♀ CC	15	0–59	12.7
DZ ♀♀ DC	7	11–113	69.3
DZ ♂♀ CC	23	0–66	16.6
DZ ♂♀ DC	21	13–130	82.9

For this reason in Table II we have examined the IQs of normal MZ twins reared apart in the four famous studies of Newman, Freeman, and Holzinger [1937], Shields [1962], Juel-Nielsen [1965], and Burt [1966] giving a total of 122 separated MZ pairs (calculated from the raw scores reported by Cronin et al. [1975]). Internal inconsistencies in these studies have been reported by several researchers [Kamin, 1974; Cronin et al., 1975]. Kamin [1974] noted that in Shields' study the separated twins were raised in the homes of relatives and friends, while in most of Burt's twin pairs, one member of each pair was raised by the biological family.

Notwithstanding these criticisms, the data from the four studies of separated twins with normal IQs may be compared with our study of MZ twins discordant for mental retardation (who may be considered as twins separated or reared apart). The 122 twin pairs with normal IQs reared apart revealed a mean IPD of 6.5 IQ points and IPDs in IQ ranging from 0 to 24 points. Twenty-six of these twins (21.3% of the 122 twins) had IPDs greater than 10 IQ points. In our study all 12 of the MZ twin pairs (100%) discordant for mental retardation (ie, reared apart) had IPDs greater than 10 IQ points.

The range and means of the IQs of twins reared apart and together are shown in Table III. In addition to the data from the normal IQ twins (discussed above), this table presents the range of within-pair differences (IPD) in IQ and the mean IPD of the MR twins. The MZ twins DC for mental retardation have a higher range of IPD in IQ (45–90) and mean IPD in IQ (64.3) than did the normal twins in the four studies. The like-sexed DZ twins discordant for mental retardation have almost the same IPD IQ (67.0) as the MZ DC for mental retardation, with a wider range of IPD in IQ (11–113). This is interesting as both genetic and environmental factors produce the differences seen in DZ twins discordant for mental retardation, while only environmental factors presumably cause the large differences in IQ observed among the MZ twins discordant for mental retardation. As expected, the unlike-sexed DZ twins DC for mental retardation have a mean and range much larger than do either the MZ or like-sexed DZ twins.

The wide range of IPD in IQ seen among the MZ twin pairs discordant for mental retardation may result from various environmental factors. These factors may affect, to a greater or lesser degree, singly born individuals with presumably "normal" IQ scores. These may include normal individuals in culturally, socially, nutritionally, intellectually, and/or emotionally nonstimulating or deprived (ie, low socioeconomic) environments. These in a sense are similar to the environments of many public and private so-called "schools" for the mentally retarded.

Another perspective on the question of the size of the range of inherited IQs in individuals is obtained by looking at the changes in IQ scores that occur in a single individual over a period of time.

TABLE II. IQs of Normal MZ Twins Reared Apart: Range and Means of IQ Intrapair Differences (IPD)

Study number	Author and date	Number of pairs	Range of IPD (IQ points)	Mean IQ IPD (points)
1	Newman, Freeman and Holzinger [1937]	19	1−24	7.26
2	Shields [1962]	38	0−22	6.82
3	Juel-Nielson [1965]	12	1−12	6.42
4	Burt [1966]	53	0−16	5.96

TABLE III. IQs of Twins Reared Apart and Together: Range and Means of IQ Intrapair Differences (IPD)

		Range of IPD in IQ (points)	Mean IPD IQ (points)	Number of pairs
		Twins reared apart		
Normal IQ: MZ[a]		0−24	6.5	122
MR: MZ	DC	45−90	64.3	12
MR: DZ SS	DC	11−113	67.0	12
MR: DZ OS	DC	13−130	82.9	21
		Twins reared together		
MR: MZ	CC	0−39	6.0	45
MR: DZ SS	CC	0−59	10.6	30
MR: DZ OS	CC	0−66	16.6	23

SS: Same sex; OS; opposite sex.

[a]Four studies combined from Table III.

Baroff [1974] reported that the usual IQ test-retest differences in the mentally retarded do not exceed 10 IQ points, and an average difference of less than 2 IQ points occurred in MR children retested after a three-year period. We believe that the IQ variations observed within each twin pair may be comparable to test-retest comparisons of single individuals. In the present study, 34.5% of the MZ pairs concordant for mental retardation have within-pair differences that are greater than 10 points. These data suggest that there is a larger range of intertest IQ differences in MR individuals than was previously suspected.

This finding gains further support from the IQ test-retest scores of MR twin individuals (MZ and DZ) observed over extended periods of time. Table IV presents some of these data. The differences in IQ scores are seen for several MR twin individuals and their co-twins. The co-twin with a normal IQ generally has a stable IQ (or possibly an increase in IQ scores over a period of time), whereas the MR

TABLE IV. Intertest Differences (ITD) in IQ for Individual Members of Mentally Retarded Twin Pairs

	CA	MA	IQ	IQ test
	1. Monozygotic (♂♂) twin pair, concordant for mental retardation. History: Negative (but clinical evidence of cranial anomaly)			
Twin A	8–0	4–2	52	Stanford-Binet
(ITD = 26)	11–0	2–10	26	
	12–1	3–9	31	
Twin B	8–0	4–2	52	Terman (S-B)
(ITD = 24)	11–8	3–6	30	
	12–1	3–10	32	
	14–4	4–0	28	
	15–11	4–8	29	
	2. Monozygotic (♂♂) twin pair, concordant for mental retardation. History: Strongly suggestive of brain injury			
Twin A	12–1	7–4	70	
(ITD = 17)	14–2	7–6	53	
Twin B	13–10	7–4	54	Stanford-Binet
(ITD = 24)	15–11	10–10	77	Wechsler-Bellevue
	3. Dizygotic (♂♀) twin, discordant for mental retardation. History: Evidence of mental retardation in sibs. Co-twin has normal IQ			
(ITD = 34)	5–6	3–9	68	Terman (S-B)
	5–7	4–6	81	Terman
	7–5	5–0	68	Stanford-Binet
	9–5	5–10	62	
	11–6	5–10	51	
	13–6	6–4	48	
	15–6	6–10	46	
	4. Monozygotic (♂♂) twin, discordant for mental retardation. History: Gross neglect (hospitalization and foundling home)			
(ITD = 33)	1–8	–	64	
	2–8	–	51	
	4–4	1–4	31	

twin's IQ characteristically decreases with the passage of time. The first two twins in Table IV (pair 1, twins A and B), MZ (♂♂), CC for mental retardation, have an intertest difference (ITD) of 26 and 24 for each twin, respectively, occurring over a three-year and a six-year period. The similarity in the degree of depression of the ITD in IQ suggests that these genetically identical twins reacted similarly to their institutional (New York State School) environment.

The next two twins (pair 2, twins A and B) were also MZ (♂♂) and CC for mental retardation. They have an ITD in IQ of 17 and 24 IQ points for each twin, respectively, over a two-year period. As was true of the previous twin pair, their seven-point difference in IQ suggests the similarity of genetically identical twins' response to a similar (institutional) environment. Twin 3, the male member of a DZ pair, DC for mental retardation, had an ITD of 34 IQ points over a ten-year period in a state institution.

Finally, twin 4, one member of a MZ (♂♂) pair, DC for mental retardation, showed a three-year ITD of 33 IQ points. The drop in IQ suggests a similarity in the effect of different institutional environments on IQ performance. The identical co-twin had an IQ of 81, although their early histories were very similar (low birthweight, hospitalization for 12 weeks, foundling home until they were 4 years old). But the co-twin went to a foster home, while the index case was admitted to an institution for the retarded when he was 3 years old. The co-twin with the low-normal IQ of 81 appeared more sickly at birth, had physical anomalies similar to the index case (umbilical hernias and incompletely descended testicles), and also had diminished reflexes. Yet there was a 50-point IQ difference between the twins, possibly reflective of the difference in environments (institutional vs foster home).

It would appear that these variations indicate the effect of an unstimulating institutional environment on the intellectual performance of MR individuals. By extrapolation, we suggest the same phenomenon may occur among individuals with "normal" intelligence (ie, non-MR) living in low socioeconomic, disadvantaged environments, which may mimic those in institutions for the mentally retarded.

The wider range of variation in intelligence test performances in the present study may be attributable to various factors, among them, differences in educational, nutritional, and emotional milieux. Most, if not all, of these differences may be environmentally precipitated, including the etiological agent(s) responsible for the severity of the disorders.

The physical separation of twins from birth or early infancy, overlaid with discordance for severe illnesses or disorders, provide data reflecting the wide range of intelligence test scores, and possibly intelligence itself, in genetically identical (MZ), compared to nonidentical (DZ), twins.

ACKNOWLEDGMENTS

I should like to thank Dr. John D Rainer of the New York State Psychiatric Institute for making the records of these twins available to me, and Dr. Gordon Allen for the use of the data in this study.

REFERENCES

Allen G, Kallmann FJ, Baroff GS, Sank D (1962): Etiology of mental subnormality in twins. In Kallmann FJ (ed): "Expanding Goals of Genetics in Psychiatry." New York: Grune & Stratton, chap 21, pp 174–191.

Baroff GS (1974): "Mental Retardation: Nature, Cause, and Management." New York: Wiley.

Burt C (1966): The genetic determination of differences in intelligence: A study of monozygotic twins reared together and apart. Br J Psychol 57:137–153.

Cronin J, Daniels N, Hurley A, Kroch A, Webber R (1975): Race, class, and intelligence: A critical look at the IQ controversy. Int J Ment Health 3(4):46–132.

Juel-Nielsen N (1965): Individual and environment: A psychiatric-psychological investigation of monozygous twins reared apart. Acta Psychiatr Neurol Scand Suppl 183.

Kamin L (1974): "The Science and Politics of IQ." Hillsdale, New Jersey: L Erlbaum Associates.

Newman HH, Freeman FN, Holzinger KJ (1937): Twins: A study of heredity and environment. Chicago: University of Chicago Press.

Shields J (1962): Monozygotic twins broupt up apart and brought up together. London: Oxford University Press.

Placental Type and Bayley Mental Development Scores in 18-Month-Old Twins

Patricia Welch, Kathryn Norcross Black, and Joe C Christian

Two recent studies have indicated that placental differences in monozygotic twins are associated with differential pair variation in intelligence.

Melnick et al [1977] found such within-pair greater variability in the 7-year-old IQ scores of dichorionic as compared to monochorionic monozygotic twins. The sample was from the Collaborative Perinatal Project (NCPP) and consisted of 89 pairs of monozygotic twins (53 monochorionic and 36 dichorionic pairs) and 177 pairs of dizygotic twins who had been administered seven subscales of the Wechsler Intelligence Test for Children. Analysis of variance showed the within-pair mean square for the white dichorionic monozygotic twins was significantly larger than for the white monochorionic monozygotic twins ($p < 0.01$). Within-pair differences between black monozygotic twins followed the same trend but were not significant. Melnick et al. also found that the white dichorionic monozygotic twins had within-pair mean squares almost identical to white dizygotic twins.

Using a subset of twins from the NCPP, Brown [1977] examined variation by chorion type in the IQ scores of 4-year-old twins who had been given the Stanford-Binet intelligence test. Subjects were 55 pairs of monochorionic and 44 pairs of dichorionic twins. Brown examined the data by means of Pearson product-moment correlation coefficients for within-pair correlations. He did not find any significant relationship between variation in the IQ scores and chorion type.

In sum, variability in intelligence in monozygotic twins of different chorion type has been found at 7 but not at 4 years of age. Monozygotic twins are presumed to have identical genotypes, and differences between them are ascribed to environmental influences. Thus any variability in behavior between two groups

Twin Research: Psychology and Methodology, pages 145—149

of monozygotic twins is of interest, not only for the study of the development of twins, but in its implications for sources of variation in singletons. We therefore decided to examine a population of younger twins of known placental type in order to determine what differences, if any, exist at this earlier developmental stage.

Subjects were 32 pairs of monozygotic twins, drawn from the Indiana University Twin Panel. Chorion type had been established by gross and microscopic placental examination. There were 20 monochorionic pairs and 12 dichorionic pairs. Zygosity of the twins was determined by blood groups (ABO, Rh, MNS, Kell, P, Duffy, and Kidd) and dermatoglyphic analysis [Reed et al, 1977]. Data were also available on race, birthweight (with the exception of one pair), and socio-economic status (SES). SES was determined by means of the occupation factor of the Hollingshead [1957] Two-Factor Index of Social Position. The second factor (education) was not used because it can distort socioeconomic placement by differentiating those at the same occupational level who are of different ages and therefore, possibly, of different average years of schooling [Haug, 1972]. Twins in this study belonged to SES classes 2 through 7. For the purposes of the present analysis, classes were collapsed to form two groups: middle and upper middle class, comprised of classes 2 through 4, which represent white collar occupations, and lower class, comprised of classes 5 through 7, which includes manual laborers, skilled and unskilled workers.

Eight pairs of twins were black, seven of them from families in the lower SES classification. Table I shows the distribution of the subjects by chorion type, social class, and race.

Subjects were seen in the home. The Mental Scale of the Bayley Scales of Infant Development [Bayley, 1969] was administered to each pair of twins by one of three female examiners who were graduate students in developmental psychology. The Bayley scale is a widely-used instrument which assesses infant development

TABLE I. 32 Twin Pairs by Chorion, SES, and Race

SES by class[a]	(N = 20) Monochorionic		Dichorionic	
	White	Black	White	Black
2	4		2	
3	5		1	
4			3	1
5	3	3	3	
6		1		1
7	2	2	1	

[a]No twins were from SES class 1.

up to an age of 30 months. It yields a raw score which can be converted to a mental development index (MDI) with a mean of 100 and a standard deviation of 16.

RESULTS AND DISCUSSION

Table II shows the means and standard deviations of the two groups for MDI, birthweight, and SES. When tested by a t test [Christian and Norton, 1977], none of the means between the groups differed significantly. Monochorionic and dichorionic monozygotic twins did not show significant differences in variability of MDI at an age of 18 months. The within-pair mean squares were larger for the monochorionic than for the dichorionic twins, but the F ratio did not reach statistical significance. The lack of significant differences in variation of MDI held when black twins were removed from the group.

The data were analyzed for birthweight differences. Analysis of variance yielded greater within-pair mean squares for monochorionic twins (F = 4.74; df 19, 12; p = 0.025; two-tailed test). This finding is in accord with that of Corey et al [1976] using 129 pairs of monozygotic twins from the same population as that from which the twins in the present study were drawn. Corey et al. found variation in birthweight within monochorionic twin pairs to be three times greater than that for dichorionic twins.

These studies of chorion type suggest that, while monochorionic twins are more variable than dichorionic twins in birthweight, the dichorionic twins are more variable than monochorionic twins in measures of intellectual functioning at an age of 7 years, but not at 4 years or 18 months.

The greater variability in birthweight for monochorionic twins may well be understood in terms of Bulmer's [1970] suggestion that there are dangers in sharing a placenta. Such differential birthweight might be expected to lead to greater within-pair variability in IQ, as a connection between birthweight and IQ

TABLE II. Means and Standard Deviations of MDI, Birthweight, and SES

	Monochorionic (N = 20)	Dichorionic (N = 12)
MDI mean	95.47	88.54
SD	13.38	14.03
Birthweight mean (N = 19)	2,471	2,567
SD	657	577
SES mean	4.35	4.50
SD	1.82	1.98

has been observed [Koch, 1966]. In our study, Pearson product-moment correlation showed birthweight significantly correlated with MDI (r = 0.37). Sameroff and Chandler [1975], in their comprehensive review of reproductive risks, suggest that low birthweight may be the most important factor in the developmental deficit typically shown in premature infants. However, they concluded that such early developmental risks did not have lasting effects, as previously thought. The organism has a "self-righting" tendency which helps it to overcome prenatal and perinatal deficits, particularly in a favorable environment. Low birthweight had an adverse effect on IQ in later development only in the lower SES groups.

The role of SES has also been clearly established as a factor in ability scores: the lower the SES, the lower the IQ. Pearson r values for our data showed SES to be significantly correlated with MDI (r = −0.37) and birthweight (r = −0.31). Whites had greater birthweights and more were in the upper SES group, and the greater the birthweight and SES, the higher the MDI. Stepwise regression showed SES to be the most important variable in relation to MDI, as it was in the NCPP study: It accounted for 0.14 of the variance. Birthweight was the second factor to emerge and accounted for 0.07 of the variance in MDI. We are offering the hypothesis that, whatever the factors which bring about the greater reported dichorionic variability in IQ at 7 years of age, they are masked in early development by the short-term effects of the differential birthweight in monochorionic twins.

It is possible that monozygotic variability according to chorion type may be a function of one stage of postnatal development and not another. The present data suggest that it is useful to continue to do research to confirm or reject the findings, with data gathered from different age groups.

SUMMARY

The mental development of 18-month-old twins was examined to determine if any differences exist in variability by chorion type. No significant differences were found in mental development between monochorionic monozygotic and dichorionic monozygotic twins. This is in contrast to the finding of Melnick el al [1977] regarding IQ variation of 7-year-old twins. Brown [1977], however, drawing from the same population as Melnick, did not find significant differences in 4-year-old twins. Our data showed significant differences in birthweight for monochorionic twins and significant correlations of birthweight and SES with MDI. Possibly birthweight and low SES are overwhelming influences on the young organism but disappear later with growth and development of the child. The importance of the prenatal environment, particularly in the earliest stages, is stressed, as is the need for further research on chorion type in relation to the twin model.

REFERENCES

Bayley N (1969): "Bayley Scales of Infant Development Manual." New York: Psychological Corporation.

Brown B (1977): Placentation effects on birth weight and IQ in MZ twins. Paper presented at the meeting of the Society for Research in Child Development, New Orleans.

Bulmer MG (1970): "The Biology of Twinning in Man." Oxford: Clarendon Press.

Christian JC, Norton JA (1977): A proposed test of the difference between the means of monozygotic and dizygotic twins. Acta Genet Med Gemellol (Roma) 26:49–54.

Corey LA, Kang KW, Christian JC, Nance WE (1974): Birthweight in MZ and DZ twins of known placenta type. Paper presented at the First International Congress of Twin Studies, Rome.

Haug M (1972): Social class measurement: A methodological critique. In Thielbar GW, Feldman SD (eds): "Issues in Social Inequality." Boston: Little, Brown.

Hollingshead AB (1957): Two factor index of social position. Unpublished manuscript.

Koch H (1966): "Twins and Twin Relations." Chicago: University of Chicago Press.

Melnick M, Myrianthopolous NC, Christian JC (1977): The effects of chorion type on variation in IQ in the NCPP twin population. Paper presented at the Second International Congress of Twins, Washington, DC.

Reed T, Norton JA Jr, Christian JC (1977): Sources of information for discriminating MZ and DZ twins by dermatoglyphic patterns. Acta Genet Med Gemellol (Roma) 26:87–88.

Sameroff AJ, Chandler JJ (1975): Reproductive risk and the continuum of caretaking casualty. In Horowitz FD (ed): "Review of Child Development Research," vol 4. Chicago: University of Chicago Press.

Twins as a Basis for the Causal Analysis of Human Personality

LJ Eaves

INTRODUCTION

It is my intention in this paper to concentrate primarily on results rather than methods, and to keep formulas to a minimum. In defense of formulas, however, it must be said that it is only when we subject our research to the discipline of mathematical formulation and statistical test that we are able to make the most powerful and effective inferences about human variation. As long as we describe only by words, we are avoiding the hard-nosed criticism of statistical analysis and are maintaining, perhaps conveniently, a position which is at best imprecise and at worst irrefutable.

An encouraging sign has been the growing recognition that we do not have to be confined by conventional experimental designs or restricted by the simple classical models applicable to the twin study. The limitation in our research into the causes of human variation should not be the mathematical expertise of the experimenter since modern computers can overcome many of the mathematical limitations of individuals by making the refinements of numerical methods more easily accessible to the relative amateur. The limiting factor should be the ingenuity of the scientist in the specification of flexible models for individual differences and in the collection of data which enable such models to be tested in practice. Providing we have the insight and imagination to specify a model, and the capacity to collect the necessary data, the complexities of numerical analysis can be conveniently consigned to the computer.

In this paper I shall consider primarily the work of myself and my colleagues in England because this forms part of a sustained attack on a problem which is nearing its completion. Many of the principles I enumerate could be quite

Twin Research: Psychology and Methodology, pages 151–174

adequately illustrated by reference to the data of others. The methods employed in data analysis are those of maximum likelihood, or methods which, asymptotically at least, yield maximum-likelihood estimates of parameters. Many of the later results of this paper are unpublished hitherto, and may still stand the test of revision in subsequent work. They have, however, been included in their preliminary form for the sake of completeness.

An important question of practical concern to those who use twins is the extent to which they provide a valid basis for our attempts to generalize about the causes of human variation. I shall illustrate with data on personality, in particular on extraversion and neuroticism as they are measured by the Eysenck Personality Questionnaire (EPQ) with its precursors and derivatives. My consideration will be devoted exclusively to differences between individuals within a population rather than differences between the means of different population or groups within a population.

There are several kinds of generalization which it is sometimes tempting to make about behavioral variation, and the extent to which such generalizations are justified will be considered in turn in the light of data on personality. Thus while shedding some light on the substantive causes of personality differences, I hope to illustrate some more general principles relevant to all research in this area which are more or less apparent to workers in the field.

I shall discuss the extent to which available data justify the following generalizations: across sexes; across occasions of testing; across tests; and across different types of relationship and different age groups.

THE TWIN DATA

Before we can entertain any generalizations, we must consider what kind of model the twin data themselves suggest for the causes of variation in personality. Table I presents some summaries of twin data, for adults and juveniles tested on the adult and juvenile versions of the EPQ [Eysenck and Eysenck, 1975]. The subjects were all self-selected to a greater or lesser extent: the adults by volunteering to participate; the juveniles by "being volunteered" by their parents. The age range of the adults is from 18 to 84 years old. The juveniles are all under 16 years old. In Table I are the mean squares obtained by conducting an analysis of variance of the twin pairs. The linear component of age regression has been extracted from the variation between twin pairs, hence the loss of an additional degree of freedom from the between-pair variation. In the case of juveniles the sample was supplemented by inclusion of a number of singletons in an attempt to increase the power of our analysis of any competitive or cooperative effects which might be present [Eaves, 1976].

TABLE I. Mean Squares for Twins and Singletons

Twin group	Item	Adults			Juveniles		
		df	extraversion	neuroticism	df	extraversion	neuroticism
MZ female	Between pairs	231	109	105	52	59	92
	Within pairs	233	40	43	54	13	37
MZ male	Between pairs	68	143	129	63	53	93
	Within pairs	70	32	43	65	14	37
DZ female	Between pairs	123	108	78	41	41	58
	Within pairs	125	75	68	43	28	23
DZ male	Between pairs	45	79	71	42	34	63
	Within pairs	47	54	62	44	34	63
DZ male/ female	Between pairs	66	75	87	80	36	96
	Within pairs	67	53	62	81	30	53
Singleton females	Variance	—	—	—	117	43	66
Singleton males	Variance	—	—	—	102	42	60

Let us consider only one of the studies in detail. The analyses of the adult scores for extraversion, for example, reveal certain salient points. The picture is fairly consistent in that the variation within dizygotic (DZ) twin pairs of all three types exceeds that within monozygotic (MZ) pairs to a comparable extent, while the variation within pairs is consistent over sexes. It thus seems as if there is indeed genetic variation for the trait and that the magnitudes of any genetic and environmental effects are approximately equal over sexes. The results are broadly similar for the other age groups and traits in the study. Such statements are crude and approximate. Is it possible to specify more precisely the kind of model which is adequate to explain the observed pattern of variation between and within twin pairs and to provide parameter estimates?

COMPARING MODELS

Table II illustrates the results of such an analysis for adult and juvenile extraversion scores. A similar analysis applies broadly to neuroticism. Table II summarizes attempts to compare alternative models for variation in extraversion. Across the table are listed a series of hypotheses which might be propounded, and down the columns are a number of plausible alternatives. Each cell of the table provides certain information basic to the discrimination between models, namely, the values of chi-square, with its associated degrees of freedom (df) and probability (P), derived from an approximate likelihood ratio test for comparing the model specified at the head of the corresponding column with that provided in the heading of the intersecting row. Thus the first cell of the first row gives the outcome of the likelihood ratio test for comparing the hypothesis that the ten mean squares reflect the influences of environmental variation within families (E_1) and the effects of additive gene action (V_A) given random mating, with the alternative that each of the ten statistics should be given its own unique value ("the perfect fit" solution). The chi-square has eight degrees of freedom because two parameters are estimated from ten statistics. The fact that the chi-square has a nonsignificant value implies that we could, with considerable parsimony, express our ten observed mean squares by reference to only two parameters and that an explanation in quite simple terms provides an adequate summary of these data. Several alternatives may be compared with the perfect fit. Typical possibilities are tabulated. The second column is related to fitting a third parameter to allow either for the presence of dominance (V_D) or for environmental differences between families (E_2). Additional variation due to assortative mating and any covariance of genetic and environmental variation between families will be confounded with E_2, and under some circumstances the effects of dominance and E_2 may cancel one another out in twins reared together. However, a marked excess of either one or the other will lead to a significant improvement in fit if a third parameter is added

TABLE II. Comparison of Alternative Models of Variation in Twins' Extraversion Scores

Alternative model	Statistic	Hypothesized model									
		Adult twins					Juvenile twins + singletons				
		V_aE_1	$+E_2/V_D$	competition	sex-limitation	E_1E_2	V_AE_1	$+E_2/V_D$	competition	sex-limitation	E_1E_2
"Perfect fit" (goodness of fit)	χ^2	11	10	10	11	31	10	5	2	8	25
	df	8	7	7	6	8	10	9	8	8	10
	P%	20	20	20	5–11	1	43	81	98	41	1
V_AE_1	χ^2	—	1	1	0	—	—	5	7	2	1
	df	—	1	1	2	—	—	1	2	2	—
	P%	—	20–30	20–30	90	—	—	2–5	2–5	30–50	—
E_1E_2	χ^2	—	22	22	21	—	—	21	22	17	—
	df	—	1	1	2	—	—	1	2	2	—
	P%	—	1	1	1	—	—	1	1	1	—
E_1 ("chance effects")	χ^2	95	96	96	95	75	36	41	43	38	21
	df	1	2	2	3	1	1	2	3	2	1
	P%	1	1	1	1	1	1	1	1	1	1

to the model. We see that the three-parameter model does indeed fit the data, which is not surprising, since we had already shown that the more restricted $V_A E_1$ model is sufficient. Comparing the model with the reduced model, however, by inspecting the results of the second cell on the second row of Table II, confirms that the additional parameter does not yield a significant improvement in the likelihood of obtaining the observed mean squares. Instead of specifying either V_D or E_2, it is possible to consider a simple model for competitive or cooperative effects [Eaves, 1976a], which allows for the influence of the genotype of one twin upon the phenotype of the other, by specifying the contribution of the "genetic environment" to environmental variation and to the covariation of genes and environment. Such a model fits the data (line 1, column 3, of Table II), but does not improve the fit significantly over that obtained for the $V_A E_1$ model (line 2). In the initial cursory examination of the mean squares it was suggested that the effects of genes were consistent over sexes. The fourth column summarizes tests of this hypothesis by permitting the expression of gene action to depend on sex. The model allows the genetic variance to be unequal in the two sexes, and the correlation between gene effects in males and females to be less than unity. The model employed is discussed by Eaves [in press], and from Table II can be seen to provide little improvement over the initial $V_A E_1$ model. If genetic effects are deleted entirely from the model such that only E_1 and E_2 components are specified (column 4 of Table II), we see that the model gives a fit which is significantly poorer than the perfect fit, implying that such a reduction is not justified by the data. On the other hand, models which involve some form of gene action, in the form of additive effects, competition, or sex limitation, give a significantly better fit than models which assume only E_1 and E_2 (row 3 of Table II) while all the models, including the $E_1 E_2$ model, yield a significantly better fit than that which assumes all the variation is due to environmental differences within families (row 4). Thus, if we are prepared to adopt Occam's razor and accept the simplest model which provides an adequate fit for the observations, we would be compelled to adopt as our working model the view that all the variation in extraversion is attributed to the additive effects of genes and environmental differences within families.

Further examination of the results in Table II shows broadly the same picture for extraversion in juveniles, although it could now be argued that the $V_A E_1$ model is not entirely satisfactory since a marginally significant improvement is obtained if allowance is made for competition or dominance. This possibility will be examined in more detail subsequently.

PARAMETER VALUES

In Table III the actual parameter estimates are given for adult extraversion and neuroticism scores for two models. In both cases the chi-square testing goodness-of-fit is not significant for the simple $V_A E_1$ model, and in both cases somewhat less than half the total variation is apparently due to additive genetic effects. The consequences of allowing for dominance are also illustrated. There is no marked improvement in fit for either trait, but the standard errors of V_A and V_D show a sharp increase. This is due to a correlation of the order of -0.9 between estimates of V_A and V_D and reveals the considerable weakness of the twin design for resolving additive and nonadditive genetic effects. The large negative correlation between the estimates also explains the negative (but not significant) value of V_A for neuroticism. Table III reveals in a very simple way the limits of the twin design for the resolution of different kinds of gene action. The correlations between estimates of additive and dominance variation are very marked, with the result that, although there are manifest genetic effects (reflected in the joint significance of V_A and V_D), it is very difficult to identify the effect of dominance unambiguously except when the heritability is high and the dominance ratio large [Eaves, 1972; Martin et al, in press].

SEX INTERACTION

Earlier it was stated that there was no evidence that the expression of genetic differences depended on sex. The basis of this statement was the fact that allowance for such interaction of genetic differences with sex did not lead to a significant improvement in fit. Table IV makes this more explicit by considering the consistency of gene expression over sex for extraversion and neuroticism in adults. The parameters V_{AM} and V_{AF} are the additive genetic variance in males and females, respectively. The critical parameter for the assessment of the consistency of gene expression over sexes, however, is V_{AMF} which is the covariance between the additive effects of genes in males with their effects in females. The precise specification of this model is given in Eaves [in press]. The important point is that this parameter can be only estimated when related pairs of unlike sex are included in the study. The view

TABLE III. Parameter Estimates for Adult Twins

Parameter	Trait			
	extraversion		neuroticism	
V_A	39 ± 4	16 ± 23	31 ± 4	-19 ± 112
V_D	–	24 ± 24	–	34 ± 12
E_1	40 ± 3	39 ± 4	44 ± 3	42 ± 19
x^2	10.96	9.53	5.25	2.36
df	8	7	8	7
P%	20	20	70	90

TABLE IV. Consistency of Gene Action Over Sexes

	Extraversion	Neuroticism	Risk-taking
V_{AM}	37	39	22
V_{AF}	40	30	28
V_{AMF}	33	26	1
r_{AMF}	0.86	0.76	0.03

that twin studies should involve only pairs of the same sex in what amounts to an attempt to "control" for sex is in my view entirely misguided because the critical control group is therefore deliberately omitted from the study. In Table IV the covariance of gene effects between the sexes has been converted for convenience into a correlation r_{AMF} which may be crudely conceived as an estimate of the proportion of genes which are expressed in both sexes. For extraversion and neuroticism the proportion is fairly high. Since in neither case was the inclusion of sex limitation of this type associated with a significant improvement in fit, we must assume that r_{AMF} cannot be shown to differ significantly from unity. That is, within the limits of our study, there is no reason to suppose that different loci are being expressed in the two sexes. Just to show that this is not necessarily the case, Table IV also includes the same components for a measure of risk-taking which may be regarded as a primary factor of impulsiveness and thus contributes indirectly to extraversion. In this case there is significant additive genetic variation (as measured by V_{AM} and V_{AF}) in the two sexes, but inclusion of the unlike-sexed pairs in the analysis reveals that there is almost no communality of gene expression in the two sexes. There is no reason to suppose that any of the loci contributing to variation in male risk-taking are being expressed in female risk-taking, and vice versa. A mere comparison of the heritability estimates for males and females would be entirely uninformative since these would be approximately equal and would yield no insight at all into the underlying fundamental difference between the sexes for the trait in question. Although this example has been conducted in the framework of a genetic model, exactly analogous models can be specified for environmental components of variation and these would require very similar techniques for their resolution. The general conclusion is simply that the inclusion of pairs of unlike sex in any family study provides a critical test of certain assumptions and may reveal some surprises.

DIRECTIONAL NONADDITIVITY

So far the inferences made have been restricted to second degree statistics since, more often than not, it is "variation" that we are attempting to explain in studies of this type. However, it has long been recognized that statistics of a higher order, though more difficult to estimate precisely, can yield some helpful information about the sources of variation which would remain undetected in the analysis of second degree statistics [Fisher et al , 1932]. In Table V some simple tests are considered for the neuroticism scale of an older questionnaire for measuring psychoticism, extraversion, and neuroticism (PEN) because they may elucidate some of the subsequent facets of this study. The intercorrelations are given for the age, mean neuroticism score, and absolute intrapair difference for pairs of MZ and DZ twins. Both types of twins show the characteristic decline of neuroticism score with advancing age [Eaves and Eysenck, 1976a]. More interesting, however, is the finding that intrapair differences for MZ twins are not linearly related to pair means. This test, proposed by Jinks and Fulker [1970] and subsequently misunderstood repeatedly, is a means simply of detecting any systematic tendency of environmental effects to depend on loci associated in location or effect with those affecting the overall expression of the trait. As such, the test is capable of detecting genotype-environmental interactions of practical significance since they are systematically related to a measurable aspect of the phenotype. The absence of such linear relationship for neuroticism scores implies that there is no justification for assuming that individuals predisposed be be neurotic, *as the trait is measured by this scale,* display any greater or lesser sensitivity to the range of environmental treatment differences they experience. The other implications of the test are considered elsewhere [Jinks and Fulker, 1970; Eaves et al., 1977]. Since this correlation is not significant, we can also discount linear relationships between measurement error and neuroticism score, and proceed with a little more confidence to consider the other correlations of the set. That between DZ means and absolute intrapair differences is not significant. This means that we have no evidence for unidirectional genetic effects, such as directional dominance, directional epistasis, and net tendency for alleles of increasing effect to be more or less frequent than those of decreasing effect. Considering, finally, the correlations of age with intrapair differences reveals significant linear relationship for DZ, though not for MZ twins. This is an indication that the expression of genetical differences in the DZ twins is age dependent. This could be due simply to changes with time in the particular combinations of genes that are

TABLE V. Sources of Directional Nonadditivity in Twins' Neuroticism Scores Correlation Coefficients (%)

Variable	MZ (df 402)		DZ (df 212)	
	pair mean	intrapair difference	pair mean	intrapair difference
Age	−25**	−02	−19**	19**
Pair mean	100	04	100	−04

**Significance at 0.01 [Based on Eaves and Eysenck, 1976a].

expressed, or it could be that the correlation of genetic and environmental influences increases as a result of increasing self-selection of environments or increasing differentiation between genotypes on the part of society. Evidence will be presented shortly which supports the former view in preference to the latter.

CAUSES OF JUVENILE VARIATION

In view of the suggestion that gene expression may depend on age, it is appropriate at this point to examine the comparability of adult and juvenile behavior from the causal viewpoint. First, the results of fitting models to the juvenile EPQ scores are considered (Table VI). The results for three models are compared for extraversion and neuroticism. The first two correspond to those given for adults in Table III. The third involves, in addition to V_A and E_1, two parameters to allow for the reciprocal environmental effects of co-twins' genotypes (V_{AS}) and for the covariance between genotypic effects contributing to V_A and the genotypic effects contributing to V_{AS}. The genotype-environmental covariance is represented by V'_{AS}. This approach to the specification of sibling effects is described, in a superficially different notation, in Eaves [1976a]. Although V'_{AS}, the genotype-environmental covariance, can be detected with twin data alone, separation of V_A and V_{AS} requires that density be introduced as an independent variable in the experimental design. In this case, male and female singletons were included in addition to twins, providing two further variances for each trait and contributing two additional degrees of freedom to the chi-squares for testing adequacy of the models. Hence the chi-squares of Table VI are based on two more degrees of freedom than their apparent counterparts in Table III. For both extraversion and neuroticism it could be argued that the simple $V_A E_1$ model provides an adequate summary of the data. Certainly for neuroticism there is little to be gained from including either dominance (V_D) or cooperative/competitive effects based on genetic differences.

TABLE VI. Parameter Estimates for Juvenile Twins and Singletons

Parameter	Extraversion			Neuroticism		
V_A	21 ± 2	−6 ± 10	28 ± 4	28 ± 5	32 ± 19	27 ± 8
V_D	—	28 ± 10	—	—	−4 ± 20	—
E_1	16 ± 2	15 ± 2	14 ± 2	35 ± 4	36 ± 4	36 ± 5
V_{AS}	—	—	−3 ± 5	—	—	−1 ± 8
V'_{AS}	—	—	−4 ± 2	—	—	−1 ± 3
χ^2	10.09	5.30	3.07	12.63	12.74	12.80
df	10	9	8	10	9	8
P%	43	81	93	25	17	12

The results for extraversion suggest formally that an excellent fit would be obtained by allowing for additional sources of variation, though it would not be very clear from these data whether the improvement would be better explained by dominance (bearing in mind the significant estimate of V_D for the second model) or by competition (having regard to the significant and negative estimate of genotype-environment covariance in the third model). The data do suggest that the correlation for DZ twins is significantly less than would be expected on the simple additive model. This is not a novel finding for extraversion.

In the absence of any clear justification for choosing between the two alternative extensions of the model for juveniles, we will adopt, as a first approximation, the model which is, by the criterion of the goodness-of-fit test, sufficient to summarize the data and work on the assumption that gene action is additive and the environmental variation is all attributable to treatment differences within families. This assumption about the source of environmental differences is not adopted arbitrarily since the presence of substantial between-family environmental effects would lead to failure of the $V_A E_1$ model in the first instance and would yield significant negative estimates of V_D when the model was extended, mistakenly, to allow for dominance. Martin et al. [in press] consider the feasibility of detecting environmental variation between families with the simple twin study, and show more precisely the circumstances under which such effects may be detected. In none of the examples considered here is there any suggestion at all that the data were forcing an interpretation which involved between-family environmental effects. This statement will be subjected to further examination later.

RELATIONSHIP BETWEEN ADULT AND JUVENILE PERSONALITY

It now follows to ask to what extent adult personality, as measured by the EPQ, could be predicted from juvenile personality, as measured by the JEPQ. This would, of course, require a longitudinal study. However, we can ask a no less relevant question as far as development is concerned and consider the extent to which the genes contributing to juvenile personality are still expressed in the adult. We are fortunate in having, for the parents of the juvenile twins and singletons, the EPQ responses of their parents. Thus we have estimates of additive genetic variation in adults and juveniles (from the twins) and an estimate of the parent-offspring covariance from the parents and juvenile twins and singletons. In the absence of cultural effects (which would normally be detected by a significant between-family environmental component in the twin data) this covariance estimates one-half of the additive genetic covariance between adult and juvenile personality, as measured by the EPQ and JEPQ. Young [1977] employed the method of maximum likelihood to obtain efficient estimates of the parameters of such a model so that allowance could be made for the fact that each individual (in a juvenile twin family) entered into three relationships. That is, a female parent, for example, is both spouse of the male parent and mother to two twins. In Table VII estimates are given of the additive genetic variance in adults and juveniles and of the additive genetic covariance between EPQ and JEPQ measures of extraversion and neuroticism. The estimates of the within-family environmental variance (E_{1A} and E_{1J}) are also given. With the genetic variances and covariance it is possible to estimate r_{AAJ}, which is the additive genetic correlation between the EPQ and JEPQ and may be simply regarded as an approximation to the proportion of genes of which the effects on adult and juvenile personality are common to both. The results suggest that juvenile extraversion is substantially dissimilar genetically from adult extraversion, whereas the community of adult and juvenile neuroticism, as measured by these tests, is somewhat greater.

CONSISTENCY OF BEHAVIOR OVER TIME

Findings like those just cited suggest that a long-term developmental study of personality would be capable of identifying the causes of communality between occasions of measurement, and indeed the causes of occasion-specific variation. We do not have any long-term data of this type, but we are able to extract from our studies of the PEN and EPQ a small neuroticism scale which was administered to twins at a two-year interval. The full analysis of these data has already appeared [Eaves and Eysenck, 1976] but the essence is given in Table VIII, which presents the analyses of variance of the change scores for the twins over the two-year interval between administration of the PEN and EPQ. Although there was significant common variation over the two occasions [Eaves and Eysenck, 1976b], and although this appeared to have the familiar genetic basis, examination of the analysis of change suggests a different pattern. Although all the mean squares of Table VIII are significant when tested against an appropriate error term, suggesting a significant interaction of subjects and occasions of testing (ie, "real" personality changes were taking place in the inter-

TABLE VII. Covariance Between Adult and Juvenile Personality

	Extraversion	Neuroticism
V_{Aj}	18	29
V_{AA}	39	31
V_{AAj}	13	20
E_{1A}	40	35
E_{1j}	17	36
r_{AAj}	0.49	0.67

TABLE VIII. Repeatability of Neuroticism After
Two Years

Twin type	Item	df	MS
MZ_F	B	201	19
	W	202	18
MZ_M	B	50	24
	W	51	16
DZ_F	B	103	21
	W	104	19
DZ_M	B	24	23
	W	25	17
DZ_{MF}	B	58	16
	W	58	19

Tables VIII and IX modified from Eaves and
Eysenck 1976b.

vals between tests), there is very little reason to suppose that the direction and
degree of change are influenced by genetic factors, or indeed by environmental
factors shared by members of the twin pairs. This can be inferred simply from
Table VIII since there is little suggestion that the mean squares between pairs
significantly exceed those within pairs for any of the twin groups, and there is
no evidence of the effects of genetic segregation since the variation within DZ
pairs does not exceed that within MZ pairs. Thus, it appears that the factors
responsible for the short-term, significant personality changes are purely chance
environmental experiences of individual twins rather than shared familial experiences.

Studies of behavior are still, characteristically, "once-off" affairs, involving
the measurement of individuals on a single occasion. There is, however, a growing interest in profiles of behavioral measurement and the genetic analysis of
change [eg, Wilson, 1975; Dworkin et al, 1976]. Twins provide a unique
opportunity to investigate the factors which contribute to both stability and
change in human behavior, as long as the study is designed to measure change.
This simple example shows how the factors influencing overall performance
of an individual may be substantially different from those which contribute to
instability over time. Such is no new finding in quantitative genetics.

PATTERN OF INCONSISTENCY

We have dealt, in a variety of ways, with the consistency of behavior over
time. The problem I wish to consider now is the consistency of patterns of
determination over different, correlated measures. This field has abounded in
theories. There have been somewhat fewer models, and very few serious
attempts to test many of the models proposed. The kind of theory I have in

mind is the possibility that genetic and cultural effects operate on what is common to several variables, whereas specific environmental influences affect what is specific. Of course, this may be a gross oversimplification, but these are the kinds of hypotheses we would like to test. I wish to consider two approaches. The first is very simple-minded, but has the advantage of being easy. The second involves a more sophisticated multivariate approach. Both, in their respective ways, are revealing. The first approach involves the analysis of test inconsistency. Table IX presents the analysis of the interaction of the subjects' x items for the 11-item neuroticism questionnaire considered previously (Table VIII). The inconsistency mean squares are all significant when tested against the pooled three-way interaction of subjects, items, and occasions of testing. This suggests that there is significant consistency in the specific profile of "neurotic" responses to the 11 items over the two occasions of testing. The data are analyzed in more detail by Eaves and Eysenck [1976b], but a cursory examination of Table I reveals the principal characteristics of their results. In every case, the pairs' x items interaction effect is significant, implying that there are genetic or cultural differences between pairs which contribute to the response profile. Furthermore, there is a consistent and significant excess of variation in response profile in DZ pairs when these are compared with MZ pairs, suggesting that the response profile is itself affected by genetic segregation. The implication of this analysis is simple enough. Genetic factors are quite specific in their action, contributing as much to highly specific profiles of response as to overall "neurotic" predisposition. Eaves and Eysenck [1976b] estimated that about 47% of the consistent variation in subject profiles was due to genetic factors; this is quite comparable with their estimate of 59% for the overall reliable, consistent neurotic behavior as measured by this short scale and would seem to be a fairly general finding. Hewitt [1974], for example, studied the item x subject

TABLE IX. Inconsistency of 11 Neuroticism Items

Twin type	Item	df	MS
MZ_F	B	2,010	29
	W	2,020	16
MZ_M	B	500	27
	W	510	18
DZ_F	B	1,030	27
	W	1,040	22
DZ_M	B	240	27
	W	250	22
DZ_{MF}	B	580	25
	W	580	20
Pooled error			10

interactions for social attitudes and showed that, while cultural effects (augmented possibly by the genetic consequences of assortative mating) contributed to variation in subjects' radicalism scores, the specific profile of subjects' responses reflected mainly genetic influences and environmental influences within families. That is, in this case, insofar as cultural effects and the mating system are important, they contribute to the overall expression of the trait, while they do not contribute significantly to the differentiation of specific attitude profiles. The latter seem to be influenced as much by the genetic background of the individual as by the environment in which he develops.

GENERAL AND SPECIFIC TRAITS

The second approach, based by Martin and Eaves [1977] on Jöreskog's [1973] method for the analysis of covariance structures, has more appeal as a method for testing hypotheses about the basis of trait covariation. The practical application of the method is likely to be most effective with relatively small numbers of measurements chosen for explicit reasons, rather than as an exploratory device for sifting through large volumes of unreduced data. Eaves et al. [in press] illustrate the approach with data on four measures of impulsiveness devised by Sybil Eysenck [Eysenck and Eysenck, 1977]: "Impulsiveness in the narrow sense," "risk-taking," "nonplanning," and "liveliness." An earlier analysis of the components of extraversion [Eaves and Eysenck, 1975] suggested that variation in impulsiveness in twins was consistent with the simple model assuming random mating, additive gene action, and within-family environmental effects. The initial task of the multivariate analysis, therefore, was to determine whether the separate study of the components of impulsiveness was consistent with the study of Eaves and Eysenck in suggesting the same mechanism for the variation and covariation in the four traits. Starting with the five groups of twins, male and female MZ pairs, male, female, and unlike-sexed DZ pairs, we fitted a model to the covariance matrices of the five twin groups which assumed that there was a single common factor underlying the four variables. It was assumed that the factor was affected by both genetic and environmental factors in such a way that the genetic loadings could be regarded as constant multiples of the environmental loadings. It was also assumed that there were both genetic and environmental variation specific to each test. It was further assumed that any genetic effects were additive and consistent over sexes, that mating was random, and that the environmental variation within families was consistent over sexes. The method of maximum likelihood [Jöreskog, 1973] was employed, and some of the initial results are presented in Table X. The log-likelihood (plus a constant) is given for this model on the first row of the table. To provide some test of the adequacy of this model, the result was compared with the likelihood obtained by letting each variance and covariance in the original

TABLE X. Models for Structure of Impulsiveness

Model for					
loadings	specifics	L + C	χ^2	df	P%
$V_A = KE_1$	$V_A E_1$	17.1	–	–	–
$V_A \neq KE_1$	$V_A E_1$	20.4	6.6	3	9
$V_A = KE_1$	Sex-limited $V_A E_1$	25.1	16.0	4	<1
"Perfect fit"		69.4	88.5	83	32

data take its own value (the "perfect-fit" solution). The latter log-likelihood (from the fourth row on the table) is 69.4, giving a difference of 52.3 units over the initial model which involved 13 parameters. The likelihood ratio test thus yields a chi-square of 104.6 for df = 87 (there being 100 variances and covariances initially). The fit of this model is thus poor. What might improve the fit? One possibility is that the constraint that genetic loadings should be constant multiples of the environmental loadings is inappropriate. That is, perhaps a different common factor is responsible for genetic and environmental covariance. The second model in Table X, therefore, considers the change in likelihood achieved by allowing the genetic and environmental loadings to vary independently. The change in the log-likelihood is only 3.3 units for the addition of three extra parameters, yielding $\chi_3^2 = 6.6$, a barely significant change. It thus appears that the failure of our initial model is not a property of the factor structure but of the trait-specific variation or of the basic additive genotype-environmental model. It will be recalled that risk-taking, one of the variables considered in Table IV and entering into the present analysis, displayed marked inconsistency of gene action across sexes. The possibility must be considered, therefore, that the failure of the model was due to the inconsistency, across sexes, of the determination of the trait-specific components of variation. For this reason a third model was fitted which retained the constraint on the genetic and environmental loadings but allowed for complete independence of the specific genetic variances in males and females. The improvement in likelihood of 8 units over the initial model, for the addition of four parameters, yielded a highly significant χ_4^2 of 16.0. Furthermore, the model is not significantly worse than the perfect-fit model ($\chi_{33}^2 = 88.5$), suggesting that the third model gives a reasonable approximation to the observed situation. Details of the results are given in Eaves et al. [in press]. The principal conclusion is that the data are consistent with the original model of Eaves and Eysenck as far as the general factor is concerned. It appears that whatever is contributing to the common variation of impulsiveness is partly inherited in a consistent manner over sexes and contributes to the components of impulsiveness in the same way as the environmental experiences of individual twins. However, the same is not true for the trait-specific variation. There is evidence of significant heterogeneity of gene expression between males and females. This is most clearly seen in the summary presented in Table XI, which gives the maximum-likelihood estimates of the heritability of the common and specific components of impulsiveness, as measured by questionnaire. After the common factor has been extracted, it can be seen that there remains significant genetic variation for particular traits and that the heritability is fairly consistent over sexes, apart from the glaring exception of risk taking, for which there is apparently no specific genetic variation in males. It is not clear to me whether this finding should be taken with sufficient seriousness as to justify speculation about its biological significance.

In presenting this work, I have deliberately concentrated on a broad outline of the results rather than the method, which can be found in a more complete form in Martin and Eaves [1977] and Eaves et al [1977].

GENERALIZING TO OTHER RELATIONSHIPS

By far the bulk of this paper has been devoted, as befits a twin congress, to the analysis of twin data in an attempt to illustrate the diverse ways in which twins can be employed to test hypotheses about the nature of variation. Finally, I wish to go beyond twins and ask a fundamental question which must follow any program of twin research: "How far can the results and models developed on the basis of twin studies be used as a basis for generalization to the population as a whole?" I do this by presenting some initial results of a more extensive study of personality in twins, pedigrees, and adoption families conducted in collaboration with the Institute of Psychiatry. Since the results have been prepared somewhat in haste for this Congress, they should be received with some caution and may subsequently be revised. The "sample" consists entirely of volunteers and currently involves 2,469 adult subjects of whom 340 were sent to foster families at or near birth. As is widely recognized by now, data from such unbalanced pedigrees presents practical problems for statistical analysis because the same individual enters into many relationships but there is no consistent structure to the families contributing to the study. This means that the

TABLE XI. Estimated Contribution (%) of Additive Genetic Variance to Components of Impulsiveness

Trait	Females	Males
Common factor	39	
Specific		
Impulsiveness	35	38
Risk-taking	33	0
Nonplanning	33	33
Liveliness	14	14

usual approaches to analysis of balanced family data, based on the analysis of variances, correlations, or covariance matrices, are inappropriate. It is possible, however, as Lange et al [1976] have shown, to employ the method of maximum likelihood to estimate the parameters of a genotype-environmental model by maximizing the likelihood of observing the particular set of pedigrees for a given model by expressing the likelihood in terms of the raw observations and the expected means and covariance matrix of the members of the individual pedigrees. Lange et al. gives the formulation of the log-likelihood and its derivatives for models which are, essentially, linear variance-component models. In obtaining the preliminary results presented here, I have adopted their statistical formulation, but have for simplicity and generality of application adopted a minimization procedure which does not require algebraic differentiation of the log-likelihood function. This lacks much of the mathematical elegance of the approach of Lange et al., but greatly enhances the flexibility with which the method can be used in practice. One disadvantage of the method is that there is no convenient data summary which can be used as a basis for the analysis, and, as the authors themselves indicate, there is no straightforward test of the model. In fact, some kind of test could be constructed by analogy with the perfect-fit approach used above, but the approach is difficult to employ in practice because of the large number of parameters involved.

Table XII gives an idea of the structure of the data by indicating the number of possible pairwise comparisons which could be extracted from the data using the conventional approach. It must be stressed, however, that the same individual enters into a large number of relationships and so the pairs would not be inde-

TABLE XII. Correlational Pairings for Adults

Relationship	Number of pairs
Spouse	153
Parent	545
Grandparent	57
Uncle (aunt)	314
Great-uncle (aunt)	13
Sibling	418
DZ twin	229
MZ twin	314
First cousin	113
First cousin once removed	32
Foster parent	230
Foster child-natural child	36
Foster child-foster child	22
Total number of individuals	2,469
Total number of fostered individuals	340

pendent. Thus, although there are 545 pairs involving the parent offspring relationship, these will include the pairing of the same parent with all the off-spring of a multiple sibship, and many of the 57 grandparents will also contribute data on parent-offspring similarity. The results presented relate to the extra-version and neuroticism scores of the EPQ after transformation to angles to improve the approximation to normality and after correction for the signficant linear change in personality score with age. The age correction was conducted separately for males and females.

Several models were fitted by the approach suggested by Lange et al. to both extraversion and neuroticism. The results for extraversion are considered first (Table XIII). The twin data (see, eg, Tables II and III) suggested that a $V_A E_1$ model was adequate for extraversion, and this was adopted as the baseline for the full analysis. The parameter estimates obtained by maximum likelihood are given in Table III. We now consider what improvement, if any, is achieved by allowing for additional factors in the model. The addition of V_D to specify dominance (the second line of the table) yields an estimate which is numerically small and a trivial increase in the likelihood. It seems as if there is no marked genetic nonadditivity. Since the design has a number of individuals from foster families, it is possible to include a parameter to specify the effects of the family environment. There are many ways this may be done, depending on the origin of the familial environmental effects. Several authors have considered alter-natives [Rao et al , 1976; Cavalli-Sforza and Feldman, 1973; Eaves, 1976b]. In this case I included a simple additive effect which contributed solely to the similarity of individuals reared by the same parents but not to the similarity of parent and offspring. This is E_2 in Table XIII. Inclusion of E_2 in the additive model does not lead to a significant increase in the likelihood and produces an estimate of E_2 which is numerically small. This suggests that the family environ-ment makes only a slight contribution to variation in extraversion. For the sake of completeness the results of including both dominance and family environ-ments are presented and they confirm the small contribution of these sources to the total variation. The final model (the fifth row of Table XIII) allows for the possibility of an alternative form of nonadditivity, that due to the interaction of gene expression with age. Although the overall trend of personality score with age may be extracted by the regression approach, we have to recognize that there may still be interactions of age with genotype (or any other determinant of variation) which defy regression analysis. The final model represents one, albeit crude, approach to the problem. It is supposed that the covariance between two individuals of a given degree of relationship decays with increasing age difference between them. Thus the observed similarity between siblings, or between parents and offspring, will be a function of the underlying degree of genotypic similarity but the actual phenotypic similarity will be greatest for those whose genes are being expressed at similar ages. One possible function, which has desirable properties from the numerical viewpoint, is to regard the expected covariance $E_{c_{a_1 a_2}}$, between relatives measured at different ages a_1 and a_2, as a simple exponential function of the covariance expected if the individuals were measured at the same age, a_0, say. Then we could write

$$E_{c_{a_1 a_2}} = e^{-k|a_1 - a_2|} E_{c_{a_0}},$$

where a_1 and a_2 are known for each pair of subjects, $E_{c_{a_0}}$ is known from the causal theory embodied in the particular model, and k is a constant to be determined. If k is zero, then the expression of the determinants of familial similarity is not dependent on age. The consequences of larger values of k for relatives of a given age difference can be easily found by substitution once k is known. There are, naturally, a great many subtleties of this approach which will depend on precisely what is assumed to be age dependent, but in practice the simple model above should provide a starting point. It is worth noting in passing that estimation of k is possible only by returning to the original data.

Fitting k to allow for any age interaction of gene expression against the background of an overall $V_A E_1$ model for extraversion gave an estimate of 0.0009 for k and no perceptible change in the log-likelihood. Such a value of k implies only a marginal attenuation of phenotypic similarity between adult relatives with increasing age difference.

Turning finally to the first results for neuroticism (Table XIV) reveals a somewhat different picture. Here there seems to be more evidence of nonadditive variation. Inclusion of V_D, for example, produces an estimate which is numerically large and a significant increase in the log-likelihood. On the other hand, allowing for the family environment in the simplest possible way by specifying an E_2 parameter makes a little difference to the outcome, whether dominance is included or not. Thus the finding for the whole data set is consistent with the twin data alone in suggesting that the family environment does not contribute significantly to the similarity of natural and adopted siblings. Bearing in mind the heterogeneity of the sample with respect to age, an almost inevitable consequence of pedigree studies, it is appropriate to ask whether the nonadditivity assigned to dominance could be equally, or more effectively, assigned to genotype x age interaction. Indeed, the inclusion of k in the $V_A E_1$ model does improve the fit of the model significantly, though not as markedly as was true of dominance. Taking k at its face value would suggest that an absolute age difference of about 20 years would result in a 50% reduction in the similarity of relatives, compared with the similarity to be expected for relatives measured at the same age. Inclusion of both k and V_A gives the results in the last line of Table XIV. This model gives a marginal increase in the likelihood, when compared with the model which assumes k is zero, but a significant improvement over the model which includes k but lets V_D be zero. That is, inclusion of both

TABLE XIII. Maximum-Likelihood Pedigree Analysis of Extraversion

Model	V_A	V_D	E_1	E_2	K	L + C	χ^2	df	P%
V_aE_1	35	–	65	–	–	8.9	–	–	–
$V_AV_DE_1$	42	–8	67	–	–	9.4	1	1	30
$V_AE_1E_2$	31	–	65	5	–	9.4	1	1	30
$V_AV_DE_1E_2$	39	–15	69	8	–	10.4	3	2	20
V_AE_1K	31	–	65	–	9×10^{-4}	9.0	0	1	> 90

TABLE XIV. Maximum-Likelihood Pedigree Analysis of Neuroticism

Model	V_A	V_D	E_1	E_2	K	L + C	χ^2	df	P%
V_AE_1	29	–	55	–	–	1.3	–	–	–
$V_AV_DE_1$	8	28	48	–	–	7.9	13	1	< 1
$V_AE_1E_2$	28	–	55	1	–	2.5	2.5	1	10
$V_AV_DE_1E_2$	10	30	47	–5	–	8.4	1	1	30
V_AE_1K	33	–	50	–	4.25×10^{-2}	6.6	11	1	< 1
$V_AV_DE_1K$	–13	20	46	–	1.61×10^{-1}	8.6	4	1	5

k and V_D suggests that genetic nonadditivity represented by dominance in the model is somewhat more likely to account for the apparent nonadditivity in these data than the dependence of gene expression on age.

Clearly there are many analyses still required before these results can be considered in their full context. In particular, since there is no direct test of the models fitted by this approach, it is important to compare the correlations predicted for the different degrees of relationship with those obtained in practice. The results for neuroticism, especially, suggest that unusually small ancestral correlations will be found in view of the small additive genetic component reported for the data. Only when such comparisons are made, and further models fitted, can we be fairly confident that the models proposed for personality have any real validity.

What, then, may we conclude from all this? In my view it is that we must be equivocal about the generality of our findings from twin studies. The results I have presented suggest that twins can be a powerful source for initial hypothesis testing in relation to specific assumptions about the nature and consistency of genetic and environmental sources of variation. They can be exploited to shed light on the dependence of gene effects on sex, to reveal the primary sources of behavior profiles in content and time, and to analyze in some detail the structure of multiple variables. The findings suggest that genes may be highly specific in their patterns of activity, that generalization over different related measures of behavior and over different stages of development will not always be justified. Finally, the results from the family study suggest that, when we try to generalize from twins to the population at large, we may, for certain types of behavior, be due for surprises.

SUMMARY

Twin, family, and adoption data relating to extraversion and neuroticism illustrate how models for variation can be tested. The detection of genetic nonadditivity, sibling competition, genotype x age interaction, family environmental effects, and sex differences in gene action have been discussed. Multivariate extensions of the model fitting approach have been outlined. There is little indication of a family environment effect for either neuroticism or extraversion. The twin data suggest the same genetic and environmental effects operate in males and females. Inclusion of juvenile twins and their parents reveals that there are differences in gene expression for personality between adults and juveniles. Although gene action for extraversion is largely additive, analysis of all the data provides strong indications of nonadditive effects on neuroticism. These might be due to dominance (or epistasis) or genotype x age interaction.

Changes in neuroticism over a two-year period reflect environmental experiences of the individuals, but genetic factors influence the profile of specific personality characteristics of individuals.

ACKNOWLEDGMENTS

The author is supported by a program grant for psychogenetic research from the British Medical Research Council. Virtually all the data on which the paper is based were collected in collaboration with the Institute of Psychiatry, London, and the willing cooperation of Professor HJ Eysenck is gratefully acknowledged. The data collection was supported by the American Tobacco Corporation. Mr PA Young kindly made available his results for the analysis of the JEPQ and the parents of juveniles in advance of publication. I thank Professor JL Jinks and my colleagues Drs NG Martin and KA Last for discussion, and Mrs Judi Barker for secretarial assistance.

REFERENCES

Cavalli-Sforza LL, Feldman M (1973): Cultural versus biological inheritance. Am J Hum Genet 25:618–637

Dworkin RH, Burke BW, Maher BA, Gottesman II (1976): A longitudinal study of the genetics of personality. J Pers Soc Psychol 34:510–518.

Eaves LJ (1972): Computer simulation of sample size and experimental design in human psychogenetics. Psychol Bull 77:144–152.

Eaves LJ (1976a): A model for sibling effects in man. Heredity 36:205–214.

Eaves LJ (1976b): The effect of cultural transmission on continuous variation. Heredity 37:69–81.

Eaves LJ (in press): Inferring the causes of human variation. Proc R Statist Soc 140.

Eaves LJ, Eysenck HJ (1975): The nature of extraversion: A genetical analysis. J Pers Soc Psychol 32:102–112.

Eaves LJ, Eysenck HJ (1976): Genotype x age interaction for neuroticism. Behav Gene 6:359.

Eaves LJ, Eysenck HJ (1976b): Genetical and environmental components of inconsistency and unrepeatability in twins' responses to a neuroticism questionnaire. Behav Genet 6:145–160.

Eaves LJ, Last KA, Martin NG, Jinks JL (1977): A progressive approach to the analysis of non-additivity and genotype environmental covariation in human differences. Br J Math Statist Psychol 30:1–42.

Eaves LJ, Martin NG, Eysenck SBG (in press): An application of the analysis of covariance structures to the psychogenetical study of impulsiveness. Br J Math Statist Psychol 30: ·1–42.

Eysenck HJ, Eysenck SBG (1975): "Manual of the Eysenck Personality Questionnaire (Junior and Adult)." London: Hodder and Stoughton.

Eysenck SBG, Eysenck HJ (1977): The place of impulsiveness in a dimensional scheme of personality. Br J Soc Clin Psychol 16:57–68.

Fisher RA, Immer FR, Tedin O (1932): The genetical interpretation of statistics of the third degree in the study of quantitative inheritance. Genetics 17:107–124.

Hewitt JK (1974): An analysis of data from a twin study of social attitudes. MSc Thesis. University of Birmingham, England.

Jinks JL, Fulker DW (1970): A comparison of the biometrical genetical, MAVA and classical approaches to the analysis of human behaviour. Psychol Bull 73:311–349.

Jöreskog KG (1973): The analysis of covariance structures. In Krishnaiah PR (ed): "Multivariate Analysis," 3rd Ed. New York: Academic Press.

Lange KL, Westlake J, Spence MA (1976): Extensions to pedigree analysis. III. Variance components by the scoring method. Ann Hum Genet 39:485–491.

Martin NG, Eaves LJ (1977): The genetical analysis of covariance structure. Heredity 38:79–96.

Martin NG, Eaves LJ, Kearsey MJ, Davies P (in press): The power of the classical twin study. Heredity.

Rao DC, Morton NE, Yee S (1976): Resolution of cultural and biological inheritance by path analysis. Am J Hum Genet 28:228–242.

Wilson RS (1975): Twins: Patterns of cognitive development as measured on the Wechster Preschool and Primary Scale of Intelligence. Dev Psychol 11:126–134.

Young PA (1977): The causes of differences in juvenile personality. MSc Thesis. University of Birmingham, England

Determinants of Socioeconomic Success: Regression and Latent Variables Analysis in Samples of Twins

Paul Taubman

In this paper I will describe and summarize some research on the determinants of socioeconomic success that colleagues and I have undertaken with the NAS-NRC Twin Sample.[1] In this research we are interested both in controlling for unmeasured genetic endowments and family environment when estimating the interrelationships of measured variables such as schooling and earnings, and in estimating the contribution of genetic endowments and family environment to the variance of earnings and other measures of socioeconomic success.

A brief overview of the economic framework within which our studies are conducted may prove useful. In our work as in many other studies in economics, it is assumed that an individuals's real wages equal his marginal product where real wages equal the money wage rate divided by the price of goods produced and marginal product is the quantity of goods and services produced by the worker. Thus, individual differences in wages arise because of individual differences in marginal products which in turn depend upon a person's skills, characteristics, and attitudes, or in short, his "abilities."

In our model, as in much other work in economics, it is assumed that the abilities a person uses in the labor market are "produced" by combining genetic endowments with various aspects of inputs, such as schooling and parental time and affection. This model can, of course, be rewritten as the earnings phenotype equals the sum of earnings genotype and of environment. The motivation in most work in economics is to measure the impact of differences in specific aspects of the environment such as schooling on both the mean and the variance of earnings.

---

[1]These are published in Taubman [1976a, b] and Behrman et al [1977a, b], among others.

Twin Research: Psychology and Methodology, pages 175—187

The model used by economists to study earnings can be expressed as:

$$\ln Y = a + bS + dA + u, \tag{1}$$

where $\ln Y$ is the natural logarithm wages (or earnings if hours are fixed), S is years of schooling, A is the phenotype of all abilities except those produced by schooling, and u is a random variable which is assumed to be normally distributed. For the moment we will assume that A is unmeasured but that Y and S are measured, without error.

To evaluate the effect of schooling on earnings, we would like to obtain unbiased estimates of b. It can be shown that if we use ordinary least squares, the expected value of $\hat{b}$ (the estimate of b) obtained when A is not controlled is

$$E(\hat{b}) = b + df, \tag{2}$$

where f is given by the so-called auxilliary equation

$$A = fS. \tag{3}$$

Thus $\hat{b}$ will be biased if both d and f are nonzero or if unmeasured "ability" both affects income and is related to education.

One way to try to obtain unbiased estimates of b is to include measures of ability such as IQ in the analysis. But while there are numerous studies that have controlled for IQ and a few other abilities, it is impossible to know if measures of all relevant abilities have been included.

Suppose, however, we postulate that the production function for the phenotype of ability is dependent linearly on three unobserved variables:

$$A = G + N^C + N^T, \tag{4}$$

where G is an index of genetic endowments, N^C is an index of family or common environment, and N^T is an index of nonfamily or noncommon environment.

Substitution of Eq (4) into Eq (1) yields

$$\ln Y = a + bS + d(G + N^C + N^T) + u. \tag{5}$$

Suppose we order sibs randomly within a pair and calculate within-pair differences. Then, since G and N^C are the same for both members of a monozygotic (MZ) twin pair and since N^C is the same for both members of dizygotic twin pairs (DZ), the within-pair equations for MZ and DZ equations are given in

Eqs (6) and (7), respectively (note within-pair diffferences are denoted by Δ):

$$\Delta \ln Y = b\Delta S + d\Delta N^T + \Delta u, \tag{6}$$

$$\Delta \ln Y = b\Delta S + d\Delta G + d\Delta N^T + \Delta u. \tag{7}$$

Assuming ΔS is nonzero for some families, Eq (6) yields an unbiased estimate of b provided ΔS is measured without error and ΔN^T is uncorrelated with ΔS. For Eq (7) to yield an unbiased estimate, it is also required that ΔG be uncorrelated with ΔS.

Several comments are appropriate here. First the within-pair equations can be thought of as a type of co-twin control method; however, there is no guarantee that ΔN^T and ΔS are uncorrelated since we are not using an experimental design with random assignment. But, as discussed below, it sometimes is possible to test the null hypothesis that ΔN^T and ΔS are uncorrelated. Incidentally, since S is not assigned randomly, it too is a phenotype which varies in part because of genetic differences. Second, it is possible to test the null hypothesis that the within-pair equations for MZ and DZ twins are the same using an F test based on the analysis of covariance. Third, the technique depends crucially on the assumption that N^T does not interact with G. Using the test of Jinks and Fulker [1970] for certain types of interactions, this assumption is not rejected in our sample when we use the natural logarithm of earnings. Fourth, measurement error in S will cause the estimates of b to be biased towards zero and the bias will probably be much bigger in within-pair equations than in equations estimated across individuals. (See Taubman [1976b] for explanation.)

THE DATA

We have used a sample drawn from the NAS-NRC twin panel to estimate our earnings equations. The NAS-NRC twin panel consists of white male pairs (both veterans) who were born between 1917 and 1927.[2] Our sample consists of about 1,000 MZ and 1,000 DZ pairs who answered a survey circulated in 1974 when the twins were about 50 years old. The sample respondents have higher means but smaller variances for education and earnings than a nationwide random sample for the corresponding age cohort of white males. Most of these differences seem to occur because few people with less than ninth grade education or with earnings less than $1,000 answered our survey. However, correlations

---

[2]The sample construction and zygosity determination are given in Jablon et al. Further information on the panel and the sample is contained in Chapter 5 in Behrman et al [1977b].

between measured variables calculated across individuals are similar to those in nationwide random samples. Also across-twin (intraclass) correlations on measured variables are similar to those obtained in the few other twin samples with socioeconomic data and the DZ across-twin correlations are similar to across-sibling correlations.

REGRESSION RESULTS

Table I contains a summary of some sample regression results calculated across individuals and within pairs. When as in line 1 we treat all the individuals in the sample as unrelated individuals and when we control for no other variables, the coefficient on years of school is a highly significant 0.078, which is unchanged when age is added. It is worth emphasizing that numerous studies based on nation-wide random samples collected in 1960 or later yield very similar estimates of the schooling coefficient. From line 2 we see that holding constant a whole host of observed family background variables and marital status reduces the coefficient by about 10%. For those pairs where both were in the Navy, we have data on the General Classification Test which is primarily a vocabulary test and is a measure of cognitive skills. Controlling for this test and for the variables in the previous line reduces the education coefficient about 30% to 0.05 when the equation is estimated across pair averages.[3]

In line 4 we see that the estimated coefficient from the within-DZ-pair equation is a highly significant 0.059. This is about 25% less than the estimate in line 1 and intermediate between line 2 in which background and line 3 in which background plus IQ are controlled. Line 5 presents the within-MZ-pairs results. Here the coefficient on schooling plummets to (still statistically significant) 0.026, which is one-third of the estimate in line 1 and one-half of the estimate in line 3. Unfortunately this 0.026 is almost surely biased towards zero by measurement error. Yet other evidence suggests that correction for measurement error would result in a coefficient for schooling of 0.045 or less. Thus, in studying the effects of schooling on earnings, it is crucial to control for genetics and family environment. It also appears that measures of cognitive skill and certain aspects of family background provide fairly adequate controls — if the variance in measurement error in schooling is between 5 and 10% of the total variance in schooling.[4]

[3] This latter number is not affected much if adjustments are made for measurement error in the General Classification Test or for differences in schooling prior to taking the test.

[4] However, the estimate of 0.05 in line 3 would also be biased towards zero by measurement error. Thus there must be other abilities omitted from Eq (3) with the biases from omitted variables and measurement error approximately offsetting one another.

TABLE I. Coefficient on Years of Schooling in Equation for Natural Logarithm of 1973 Earnings

Equation based on	Number of observations	Coefficient on years of schooling	t Statistic on coefficient	Other variables held constant[a]
1. Individuals	3,872	0.078	32.4	None
2. Individuals	3,872	0.069	25.8	A, B
3. Navy pairs	404	0.051	5.9	A, B, C
4. Within DZ pairs	914	0.059	8.3	B
5. Within MZ pairs	1,022	0.026	3.5	B

[a]Other variables held constant: A) age, number of sibs alive 1940, father's years of schooling, mother's years of schooling, father's occupational status (Duncan Score); and the following variables which are coded as (0, 1) (dummies) raised in rural area, raised as a Catholic, raised as a Jew, born in the South; B) married in 1974; C) score on Navy General Classification Test.

VARIANCE COMPONENTS, LATENT VARIABLE MODELS

In discussing the statistical properties of the within-pair regressions, we noted that differences in noncommon environment might be correlated with differences in schooling since schooling was not assigned experimentally. It is possible to examine this issue using a latent variable, variance components model. This model will also allow us to estimate the contributions of genetics and common and noncommon environment to the variance in the natural logarithm of earnings and in the other variables in our model.

A latent variable is defined as an unmeasured variable that is related to more than one measured variable.[5,6] In a moment I will treat both genetic endowments and common environment as latent variables. But to indicate more clearly what we are doing, it is useful to consider a simpler example, which is set out in Table II. Here there are three Y values, each of which is "caused" by a systematic variable X and a random variable u. We will assume for now that the u variables are uncorrelated with the X variables and with each other. We would like to calculate the proportion of the total variance in each of the Y variables accounted for by X, eg, $a^2 \sigma_X^2 / \sigma_{Y_1}^2$. (Since we are interested in $a^2 \sigma_X^2$, we can with no loss in generality standardize $\sigma_X^2 = 1$.) If we use information on only one of the Y variables, say Y_1, we cannot make this calculation since our only observed statistic would be $\sigma_{Y_1}^2$ whose expected value is expressed in terms of two unknowns $a^2 \sigma_X^2 + \sigma_{u_1}^2$.

TABLE II. Hypothetical Latent Variable Model

$$Y_1 = aX + u_1$$
$$Y_2 = bX + u_2$$
$$Y_3 = cX + u_3$$

Expected values of variances and covariances
assuming u values uncorrelated with X and
each other

$\sigma_{Y_1}^2 = a^2 \sigma_X^2 + \sigma_{u_1}^2$	$\sigma_{Y_1 Y_2} = ab\sigma_X^2$
$\sigma_{Y_2}^2 = b^2 \sigma_X^2 + \sigma_{u_2}^2$	$\sigma_{Y_1 Y_3} = ac\sigma_X^2$
$\sigma_{Y_3}^2 = c^2 \sigma_X^2 + \sigma_{u_3}^2$	$\sigma_{Y_2 Y_3} = bc\sigma_X^2$

[5]For an excellent introduction, see Goldberger [1973].

[6]It is possible for the latent variable to cause (affect) a measured variable, to be caused by the measured variables, or to be the true construct that is imperfectly measured by the observed variable.

When as in Table II there are three Y values, the situation changes. In this case we have six observed variances or covariances which can be used to estimate the six unknowns (a, b, c, $\sigma_{u_1}^2$, $\sigma_{u_2}^2$, $\sigma_{u_3}^2$). The model now has a solution because the covariances of the Y values provide new observed statistics but introduce no new unknowns.

In our work we treat both genetic endowments and common environment as latent variables which appear in the system of equations given in Table III. Since this system is explained in detail elsewhere, only a few comments will be offered here.[7] First, the model in Table III has four genetic (G, . . ., G_3) and four environmental (N, . . . , N_3) variables, each set entering in triangular fashion to allow for the possibility that the four variables being studied are not dependent on the same genes or aspects of family environment. The way the G and N variables are entered, the coefficient on the new index in an equation indicates that there are different genetic or environmental effects for this dependent variable. There are also four random error terms (u_1, . . . , u_4).

Second, the dependent variables are related directly to one another, eg, schooling enters the occupational status and earnings structural equations. Thus, in the reduced form equations, which are obtained by substitution, more than one u value enters.[8] This causes a problem which can best be seen by referring back to the example in Table II. Note that if the u values in that example were not independent, the expected value of covariances of the Y values would also include the terms $\sigma_{u_1 u_2}$, $\sigma_{u_1 u_3}$, and $\sigma_{u_2 u_3}$, and we would have six observed statistics to solve a system with nine unknowns.

Third, the general model in Table III has more unknown parameters that can be estimated. We obtain an estimatable model by imposing a number of restrictions, some of which are not crucial and some of which are. We often, for example, assume that there is only one N variable. While this restriction does not alter the estimate of the contribution of environment to the variance of the Y values, it does mean we cannot determine if the same or different aspects of common environment affect the four Y values. Also in our work, we obtain some of our results, primarily the test of the hypothesis that N^T and S are uncorrelated, by imposing the condition that initial occupation has a zero coefficient in the fourth equation.[9]

---

[7] See Behrman et al. [1977b] for the most complete discussion.

[8] Vandenberg [1965] and Eaves and Gale [1974], among others, develop techniques similar to ours in models where the dependent variables are not directly related to one another. They do not estimate the parameters such as B and γ on the observed variables nor the genotypic correlations for DZ twins.

[9] For a further general discussion of identification of parameters in models of this class, see Chamberlain [1977]. Behrman et al [1977a, b] and Goldberger [1977] contain a discussion of the particular models we estimate.

TABLE III. Latent Variable Model*

(1) $Y_1 = S = aG + bN + u$

(2) $Y_2 = OC_i = cG + dN + eG_1 + fN_1 + gu + u_1$

(3) $Y_3 = OC_{67} = hG + jN + kG_1 + mG_2 + nN_1 + pN_2 + qu_1 + ru + u_2$

(4) $Y_4 = \ln Y_{73} = sG + tN + vG_1 + wG_2 + xG_3 + yN_1 + zN_2 + \alpha N_3 + \delta u + \lambda u_1 + \beta u_2 + u_3$

(1) $Y_1 = S = aG + bN + u$

(2) $Y_2 = OC_i = c'G + d'N + eG_1 + fN_1 + gS + u_1$

(3) $Y_3 = OC_{67} = h'G + j'N + k'G_1 + mG_2 + n'N_1 + pN_2 + qOC_i + rS + u_2$

(4) $Y_4 = \ln Y_{73} = s'G + t'N + v'G_1 + w'G_2 + xG_3 + y'N_1 + z'N_2 + \alpha N_3 + \beta OC_{67} + \gamma S + u_3$

where

$$c = c' + ag \qquad\qquad s = s' + \beta h + \gamma a$$
$$d = d' + bg \qquad\qquad t = t' + \beta j + \gamma b$$
$$h = h' + ra + qc \qquad v = v' + \beta k$$
$$j = j' + rb + qd \qquad w = w' + \beta m$$
$$k = k' + qe \qquad\qquad y = y' + \beta n + \gamma b$$
$$n = n' + qf \qquad\qquad z = z' + \beta p$$
$$\qquad\qquad\qquad\qquad\quad \delta = \gamma + \beta r$$
$$\qquad\qquad\qquad\qquad\quad \lambda = \beta q$$

*S is years of schooling, OC_i is occupational status in initial civilian occupation, OC_{67} is occupational status in 1967 occupation, and $\ln Y_{73}$ is natural logarithm of earnings in 1973.

Tables III–VI reprinted from Behrman, Taubman, Wales [1977a] with permission.

The reduced form of Eq (1) in Table III can be rewritten as

$$S = aG + E,$$

where $E = bN + u$. In this form and with "a" normalized to 1, the model is the one often employed in heritability studies for a single phenotype. As is well known, estimates of relevant parameters can only be obtained by making some strong assumptions. Put another way, the model is under-identified. Vandenberg [1965],, Eaves and Gale [1974], and we have shown that it is possible to test some of these assumptions, by estimating parameters for a system of equations using the individual and the MZ and DZ cross-twin variance, covariance matrices. In our work, we use a likelihood ratio test to examine the following types of restrictions. Is the only part of environment that is latent that which is common to both members of a twin pair? Is the genotypic correlation for DZ twins 0.5? Also, in principle we should be able to test whether σ_{GN} is zero though we have never been able to obtain convergence in our nonlinear maximum likelihood routine. In general, we *cannot* test the assumption that the correlation in brother's environments is the same for MZ and DZ twins.

Based on our tests, we conclude that average genotypic correlation for DZ twins for our four Y variables is about 0.35,[10] and that the only environmental variable that is latent across equations is common environment. Put another way, if $N = N^C + N^T$, we find that N^T does not enter directly into the structural equations for more than one Y.

What we consider to be our best set of equations is given in Table IV. The total effect of schooling on ln Y_{73}, which is given by the coefficient on u in the reduced form equations, is 0.026, or nearly identical to the estimate obtained from the MZ within equation. While I have not presented them here, the estimates of the coefficients on the other observed variables are also nearly identical using either the MZ within-pair regressions or the latent variable technique.

Table V contains estimates when we allow there to be four latent environmental variables and no genetic variables. This model yields estimates on the observable variables similar to the estimates in Table IV. The model in Table V fits the data less well than the model in Table IV, but Table V has fewer parameters and is not nested in Table IV; thus, a definitive statistical test of significance is not available.

Table VI contains the analysis of variance estimates based on Table IV. We find that genetics accounts for from 29 to 45% and common environment 12 to 41% of the variance in our four variables. If we assumed there were no genetic effects, then common environment would account for the sum of the G and N terms in Table VI. If we restrict the genotypic correlation for DZ twins to be 0.5, the genetic effects would be larger by about 20% and the N terms correspondingly lower.

---

[10] This coefficient is denoted λ in Table IV.

TABLE IV. Basic Four Indicator Model With λ 1/2 (24 parameters)

	G_1	N_1	G_2	G_3	G_4	u_1	u_2	u_3	u_4	S	OC_i	OC_{67}
Reduced form equations												
S	1.85 (15.9)	1.98 (17.5)				1						
OC_i	0.68 (5.5)	1.16 (11.7)	1.16 (18.5)			0.21 (6.0)	1					
OC_{67}	0.69 (6.5)	0.78 (8.4)	0.37 (5.1)	0.82 (13.8)		0.29 (8.9)	0.14 (5.4)	1				
$\ln Y_{73}$	0.17 (5.9)	0.19 (7.7)	0.098 (6.0)	0.019 (0.8)	0.31 (26.2)	0.026 (3.4)	0.0044 (3.5)	0.031 (4.7)	1			
Structural equations												
S	1.85 (15.9)	1.98 (17.5)				1						
OC_i	0.30 (1.9)	0.75 (5.7)	1.16 (18.5)				1			0.21 (6.0)		
OC_{67}	0.113 (0.1)	0.090 (1.0)	0.20 (2.3)	0.82 (13.8)				1		0.26 (7.9)	0.14 (5.4)	
$\ln Y_{73}$	0.12 (3.3)	0.13 (5.2)	0.087 (5.2)	-0.0068 (0.3)	0.31 (26.2)				1	0.016 (2.3)		0.031 (4.7)

Other estimates

$\lambda = 0.34$ (6.1): $\sigma_{u_1}^2 = 2.17$ (22.6): $\sigma_{u_2}^2 = 2.75$ (24.4): $\sigma_{u_3}^2 = 2.45$ (25.1): $\sigma_{u_4}^2 = 0.127$ (23.1)

Normalizations and Restrictions

A, B, C, D, E, F, G

Functional value = −13,431.87

Normalizations and restrictions: A is $\sigma_{G_1}^2 = \sigma_{G_2}^2 = \sigma_{G_3}^2 = \sigma_{G_4}^2 = \sigma_N^2 = 1$: B is $\sigma_{N_2}^2 = \sigma_{N_3}^2 = \sigma_{N_4}^2 = 0$: C is $\sigma_{N_1|G_1} = 0$: D is $\sigma_{N_1|G_1} = \sigma_{G_1|G_1} = 0$: E is $\sigma_{N_1|N_1} = \sigma_{G_1|G_1} = 0, i = 1,\ldots, 4$: F is $\rho' = \rho^* = 1$, where ρ' and ρ^* are the cross-twin correlations on the environments that are latent for DZ and MZ twins respectively: G is $\lambda_i = 1/2, i = 1,\ldots, 4$. The figures in parentheses underneath the point estimates are absolute values of t statistics. S is years of schooling: OC_i is initial full-time civilian occupational status, Duncan Scale: OC_{67} is occupational status in 1967, Duncan Scale: and $\ln Y_{73}$ is the natural logarithm of 1973 earnings.

TABLE V. A Pure Environmental Variable Model (21 parameters)*

	N_1	N_2	N_3	N_4	u_1	u_2	u_3	u_4	S	OC_i	OC_{67}
Reduced form equations											
S	2.76 (31.5)				1						
OC_i	1.36 (23.2)	1.17 (18.8)			0.095 (0.9)	1					
OC_{67}	1.07 (20.8)	0.34 (5.2)	0.79 (12.3)		0.26 (5.4)	0.15 (5.3)	1				
$\ln Y_{73}$	0.26 (20.1)	0.09 (5.0)	0.026 (11.2)	0.30 (19.3)	0.0053 (0.2)	0.0042 (3.1)	0.029	1			
Structural equations											
S	2.76				1						
OC_i	1.10	1.17				1			0.095		
OC_{67}	0.179	0.17	0.79				1		0.25	0.15	
$\ln Y_{73}$	0.24	0.08	0.003	0.30					-0.0021	0.15	0.029

Other estimates

$\sigma_{u_1}^2 = 1.75$ (4.2); $\sigma_{u_2}^2 = 2.73$ (16.11); $\sigma_{u_3}^2 = 2.51$ (24.3); $\sigma_{u_4}^2 = 0.129$ (13.5); $\rho^* = 0.94$ (14.9); $\rho' = 0.61$ (18.84)

Normalizations and restrictions

C, D, E, and $\sigma_{N_1}^2 = \sigma_{N_2}^2 = \sigma_{N_3}^2 = \sigma_{N_4}^2 = 1$

Functional value = -13,447.27

*Notation as in Table IV.

TABLE VI. Sources of Variance of Schooling, Initial and Later Occupational Status and Earnings (assuming $\sigma_{N_1 G_1} = \sigma_{N_1 G_1'} = 0$)*

Percentage of total arising from	S	OC_i	OC_{67}	$\ln Y_{73}$
$\sigma_{G_1}^2$	36	8	11	10
$\sigma_{G_2}^2$		23	3	3
$\sigma_{G_3}^2$			15	a
$\sigma_{G_4}^2$				32
$\Sigma \sigma_{G_i}^2$	36	31	29	45
$\sigma_{N_1}^2$	41	22	13	12
$\sigma_{u_1}^2$	23	2	4	1
$\sigma_{u_2}^2$		46	1	a
$\sigma_{u_3}^2$			53	1
$\sigma_{u_4}^2$				42

*Source: Table IV; $\lambda = 0.34$, $\rho^* = \rho' = 1$.
a) Less than 0.5%. Totals may not add to 100% because of rounding.

CONCLUSIONS

In our work we find that if one wishes to estimate the effects of changes in measured aspects of the environment or of phenotypes it is very important to control for genetic endowments and family environment. Such control can be accomplished either using within-pair regressions for MZ twins or latent variable, variance components models. At least in our work, comparable results are obtained from either method though more assumptions can be tested using the latent variable technique. The latent variable model also allows more assumptions to be tested in the analysis of variance. It also appears that for our problem the General Classification Test and certain measurements of family background provide adequate controls when estimating the coefficient of schooling but are inadequate to measure the contribution of genetics and common environment to the variance of earnings.

Since our substantive findings are based on one sample (at one point in the individual's life cycle), our results should be treated with caution. Yet we find that the extra earnings derived from education are much smaller than in other studies which have not controlled for genetic endowments and family environment. We also find that about 57% of the variance in the natural logarithm of earnings is attributable to the family, with a division between genetics and family environment of 45 and 12%, respectively. These last figures do not tell us, of course, what would happen to the mean earnings level if we changed environment. They also do not indicate that we cannot change inequality in income since we can always transfer money. But the family environment estimate is indicative of the amount of inequality attributable to inequality of opportunity (exclusive of discrimination). Thus, even with complete equality of opportunity, inequality of outcomes would be reduced by only 12%.

ACKNOWLEDGMENTS

The research summarized in this paper has been supported by several grants from the NSF and from the Hoover Institution. The project has benefitted enormously from criticism and comments of Professors Chamberlain, Goldberger, Griliches, Haspel, Jencks, and Olneck. The author is a Professor of Economics at the University of Pennsylvania.

REFERENCES

Behrman J, Taubman P, Wales T (1977a): Controlling for and measuring the effects of genetics and family environment in equations for schooling and labor market succes. In Taubman P (ed): "Kinometrics: The Determinants of Socioeconomic Success Within and Between Families." Amsterdam: North Holland.

Behrman J, Taubman P, Wales T, Hrubec Z (1977b): Inter and intra generational determinants of socioeconomic success: Genetic endowments, family and other environments. Mimeo, Economics Dept, Univ of Pa.

Chamberlain G (1977): An instrumental variable interpretation of identification in variance components and mimic models. In Taubman P (ed): "Kinometrics: The Determinants of Socioeconomic Success Within and Between Families." Amsterdam: North Holland.

Eaves L, Gale J (1974): A method for analyzing the genetic basis of covariation. Behav Genet 4:253–267.

Goldberger A (1973): Structural equation models: An overview. In Goldberger A, Duncan O (eds): "Structural Equation Models in the Social Sciences." Amsterdam: Seminar Press.

Goldberger A (1977): Twin methods: A skeptical view. In Taubman P (ed): "Kinometrics: The Determinants of Socioeconomic Success Within and Between Families." Amsterdam: North Holland.

Jablon S et al. (1967): The NAS-NRC Twin Panel: Methods of construction of the panel, zygosity diagnosis and proposed use. Am J Hum Genet, p 133–161.

Jinks JL, Fulker DW (1970): Comparison of the biometrical, genetical, MAVA, and classical approaches to the analysis of human behavior. Psychol Bull 73(No. 5, May, 1970):311–349.

Taubman P (1976a): The determinants of earnings: Genetics, family, and other environments. Am Econ Rev 66:858–870.

Taubman P (1976b): Earnings, education, genetics and environment. J Hum Resources, 11:447–461.

Vandenberg S (1965): Multivariate analysis of twin differences. In Vandenberg S (ed): "Methods and Goals in Human Behavior Genetics." New York: Academic Press.

An Examination of Fundamental Assumptions of the Twin Method

RC Elston and CE Boklage

For the purposes of this paper we shall assume we have just two samples: a sample of presumed monozygotic (MZ) twins and a sample of presumed dizygotic (DZ) twins. We shall assume these are random samples from some population, and so we need not concern ourselves here with the extra problems involved when twin pairs are ascertained via probands. We shall also restrict ourselves to the case where a single univariate measurement, x, is available on each individual in the sample. In this way we can concentrate on the fundamental assumptions underlying all twin studies, rather than the particular assumptions underlying special cases. We shall take as our purpose to estimate the heritability, or the genetic variance, of x in the population from which the twins were sampled; we can test hypotheses about a parameter if and only if that parameter is estimable. Usually x will be a continuous random variable, but this is not essential; we shall assume that x has finite mean and variance.

There are many different ways of presenting the underlying model and assumptions; we shall use the notation of Haseman and Elston [1970]. The observed values on the j-th twin pair are taken to be

$$x_{1j} = \mu + g_{1j} + e_{1j},$$

(1)

$$x_{2j} = \mu + g_{2j} + e_{2j},$$

where μ is the overall population mean, and g_{1j} and e_{1j} are the genetic and environmental effects, respectively. Over the whole population, g_{1j} and e_{1j} have zero means and variances σ_g^2 and σ_e^2, respectively.

Twin Research: Psychology and Methodology, pages 189—199

The genotypic variance σ_g^2 can be partitioned into an additive component (σ_a^2), a dominance component (σ_d^2), and an epistasis component (σ_i^2). (See, eg, Li[1976] for details of this partitioning.) It then follows from genetic principles that

$$\text{for MZ twins: } \text{Cov}(g_{1j}, g_{2j}) = \sigma_g^2,$$

$$\text{and for DZ twins: } \text{Cov}(g_{1j}, g_{2j}) = \tfrac{1}{2}\sigma_a^2 + \tfrac{1}{4}\sigma_d^2 + f(\sigma_i^2),$$

where $f(\sigma_i^2)$ refers to fractions of certain components of σ_i^2 (Cockerham [1954] give details of these components).

There are no general principles that can be used concerning the environmental effects, but for simplicity we shall assume that

$$\text{Cov}(g_{1j}, e_{1j}) = \sigma_{ge}$$

does not depend on whether the twins are MZ or DZ. For DZ twins, we define

$$\text{Cov}(g_{1j}, e_{2j}) = \text{Cov}(g_{2j}, e_{1j}) = \sigma_{ge}^{*}.$$

(For MZ twins $g_{1j} = g_{2j}$, so this quantity is then automatically σ_{ge}.)

The covariance between the e_{ij} might depend upon whether the twins are MZ or DZ, so we let

$$\text{for MZ twins: } \text{Cov}(e_{1j}, e_{2j}) = C_{MZ}$$

$$\text{and for DZ twins: } \text{Cov}(e_{1j}, e_{2j}) = C_{DZ}.$$

Finally, we make the reasonable assumption that individuals not in the same pair are independent with respect to genetic and environmental effects, ie,

$$\text{Cov}(e_{ij}, e_{i'j'}) = \text{Cov}(g_{ij}, e_{i'j'}) = \text{Cov}(g_{ij}, g_{i'j'}) = 0;$$

$$i = 1, 2; \quad i' = 1, 2; \quad j \neq j'.$$

There are various ways of estimating σ_g^2 and σ_e^2 [and hence the heritability, $\sigma_g^2/(\sigma_g^2 + \sigma_e^2)$], but they can mostly be based on the following statistics, obtained on performing among- and within-pair analyses of variance on the two types of twins:

the mean square among MZ pairs, $M_{A(MZ)}$,

the mean square within MZ pairs, $M_{W(MZ)}$,

the mean square among DZ pairs, $M_{A(DZ)}$,

the mean square within DZ pairs, $M_{W(DZ)}$.

Haseman and Elston [1970] suggest the unweighted least squares estimates

$$\hat{\sigma}_g^2 = M_{A(MZ)} - M_{W(MZ)} - M_{A(DZ)} + M_{W(DZ)}$$

and

$$\hat{\sigma}_e^2 = \tfrac{1}{4}(-3M_{A(MZ)} + 5M_{W(MZ)} + 5M_{A(DZ)} - 3M_{W(DZ)}), \tag{2}$$

which have expectations (under our model):

$$E(\hat{\sigma}_g^2) = \sigma_g^2 + \tfrac{1}{2}\sigma_d^2 + \sigma_i^2 - 2f(\sigma_i^2) + 4(\sigma_{ge} - \sigma_{ge}^*) + 2(C_{MZ} - C_{DZ})$$

and   (3)

$$E(\hat{\sigma}_e^2) = \sigma_e^2 - \tfrac{1}{2}\sigma_d^2 - \sigma_i^2 + 2f(\sigma^2) - 2(\sigma_{ge} - 2\sigma_{ge}^*) - 2(C_{MZ} - D_{DZ}).$$

It should be noted that the variance of x_{ij} is

$$\sigma_x^2 = \sigma_g^2 + \sigma_e^2 + 2\sigma_{ge},$$ (4)

and this is estimated unbiasedly by $\hat{\sigma}_g^2 + \hat{\sigma}_e^2$ as given in Eq (3) without any further assumptions. But this method of estimation can give an unbiased estimate of σ_g^2 (or a consistent estimate of heritability in the broad sense) if and only if we assume

$$\tfrac{1}{2}\sigma_d^2 + \sigma_i^2 - 2f(\sigma_i^2) + 4(\sigma_{ge} - \sigma_{ge}^*) + 2(C_{MZ} - C_{DZ}) = 0; \quad (5)$$

for this it is sufficient, but not necessary, to assume: I) $\sigma_i^2 = 0$, II) $\sigma_d^2 = 0$, III) $\sigma_{ge} = \sigma_{ge}^*$, and IV) $C_{MZ} = C_{DZ}$.

Haseman and Elston [1970] also suggest weighted least squares estimates, needing an iterative solution, and the same four assumptions are sufficient for this estimate of σ_g^2 to be unbiased. Furthermore they point out that the simple estimate

$$\hat{\sigma}_g^2 = 2(M_{W(DZ)} - M_{W(MZ)})$$ (6)

is a maximum likelihood estimate, assuming normality, if information on only the twin pair differences is available; the expected value of this estimate is exactly the same as that given in Eq (3), under the model we have assumed, and so requires the same assumption. Recently Taubman [1976] has shown how estimates can be made of bounds on heritability. Although it may appear that very few assumptions are made, restrictive assumptions similar to III and IV are in fact made; the fact that some of the assumptions are stated as inequalities rather than equalities, thus leading to estimated bounds, does not really make the critical assumptions more plausible.

Now Christian et al [1974] have considered the possibility that the variance of e_{ij} is not the same in MZ and DZ twins. They point out that the estimate of σ_g^2 given by Eq (2) is not affected by the fact that e_{ij} has a different variance between MZ and DZ twins, its expectation still being as given in Eq (3). [Their estimate $\hat{G}_{CT}$ is equal to half the estimate given by Eq (2).] They therefore recommend that this estimate be used whenever there is evidence that the variance of x_{ij}, σ_x^2, differs between MZ and DZ twins, on the assumption that such a difference is caused by a difference in variance of e_{ij} between MZ and DZ twins. But it is clear from Eq (4) that there is more than one reason why σ_x^2 might differ between MZ and DZ twins. Nance [1976] points out that the difference can reasonably be caused by a difference in σ_g^2 between MZ and DZ twins, and considers that "even if the total genetic variances are not equal, the ratio of the within-pair variance of DZ to MZ twins remains a valid test for the presence of a genetic effect in DZ twins." This is based on the fact that expectation of the estimate given by Eq (6) is as given in Eq (3) with the first four terms being the components of genetic variance *in the DZ twins* — the corresponding components in MZ twins do not enter into the expectation. But it is clear from Eq (3) that it is dangerous to conclude much from the estimate of Eq (6), which not only includes in its expectation the term $2(C_{MZ} - C_{DZ})$ but also assumes that σ_e^2 is the same for both types of twins.

Christian et al [1977] have responded to Nance pointing out that the estimate of σ_g^2 in Eq (2) at least is not biased by differences in σ_e^2, which is true. But they go on to suggest that if μ, the mean of x_{ij}, is the same in both kinds of twins, this implies that σ_g^2 is the same in both kinds of twins. Although this may be true in certain cases, it is implausible as a general rule. The simple fact is that the means and variances (and, indeed, even higher moments) can differ between MZ and DZ twins, and between twins and singletons, for either genetic or environmental reasons (or both). There are several considerations which should make this possibility obvious, as follows:

1) Dizygotic twinning is reasonably well demonstrated to have a hereditary component, the mechanism of which is assumed, but by no means proven, to be an inherited tendency to double ovulation. Monozygotic twinning is generally considered, though lately with some doubt, to have no hereditary basis. If some hereditary basis is found, it will most likely be a different one, because clearly different stages of the developmental process are affected. Given that dizygotic twins represent a different gene pool with respect to at least this one factor, it cannot be safely assumed that they represent the same gene pool with respect to any other factor.

2) A majority of MZ pairs (90% of monochorionic pairs, thus over 60% of all MZ pairs) experience some degree of fusion of placental circulations [Strong and Corney, 1967]. The phenomenon varies in its effects from none observable to the presence of the transfusion syndrome in about 15% of MZ pairs. Depending primarily on whether it is more or less evenly reciprocal or undirectional, this phenomenon may either reduce or increase within-pair variance in traits related to circulating factors such as hormones, nutrients, and waste products. Such effects have been observed in cord-blood cholesterol levels [Corey et al, 1976]. Birthweight represents a situation where both mean and variance change with chorionicity [Bulmer, 1970].

3) Twins of both zygosities are about twice as often lefthanded as are singletons. Differences across zygosities are small, but significant, in some large samples [Boklage, 1977a]. The parents of both zygosities of twins are about twice

as often lefthanded as are their own like-sexed siblings [Boklage, unpublished].
Beginning with clues provided by handedness, Boklage [1977a,b] has argued at
some length, that schizophrenia is not the same clinical entity across twin zygosity. A host of other features of mental development share with schizophrenia
the involvement of brain asymmetry development. In many respects MZ and DZ
twins are not the same kind of people, and neither group is the same as singletons,
in at least some of these features.

Thus the most fundamental assumption that is always made when we attempt
to estimate heritability from twins is that the twins, both MZ and DZ, have the
same genotypic and environmental variances as the population of singletons for
which we wish our estimates to be relevant. [As indicated above, however, it is
possible by using Eq (6) to make no assumptions about the genetic variance in
MZ twins.] There is good evidence in at least some cases that this assumption
does not hold, and there is no completely satisfactory way of testing whether it
holds in a given case. We also need to assume Eq (5), or something similar, depending on how precisely we wish to define the genetic component of variance;
the most critical part of this assumption is satisfied by III) $\sigma_{ge} = \sigma_{ge}^{*}$ and IV)
$C_{MZ} = C_{DZ}$, given above. Here again, there is no way of testing this assumption.

There are other assumptions that must be mentioned. It should be noted that
we have assumed no genotype-environment interaction in the model (1), and the
effect of such an interaction on any estimates will be dependent on the nature of
the interaction. Although it may be plausible that any interaction effect will usually be small compared to the main effects g and e, there is no general test for
interaction in the usual twin data. Certain types of interaction can lead to a relationship between the (absolute) twin pair difference and the twin pair mean
[Jinks and Fulker, 1970], but such a finding may merely be indicative of hetero-
scedasticity [Morton, 1974]. Whatever its cause, such a relationship can often be
eliminated by an appropriate transformation of the data (eg, by a power transformation of the form $y = x^{p}$).

Finally, we want to point out that the twin method assumes there are just
two types of twins, MZ and DZ, and that we know which are which. We shall
not dwell here on the problem of determining whether a pair of twins is MZ or
DZ, for which there is now a standard methodology [Gaines and Elston, 1969].
We do wish to stress, however, that no one has in fact established whether or not
a third type of twin, dispermic monovular twins, also exists.

We know that some multiple births developed from a single zygote [cf Corner,
1955]. The rest come from more than one zygote. It has been plausibly assumed
that N zygotes must represent N sperm and N ova, the latter having developed
from N primary oocytes from N follicles. It is true, in the vast majority of cases
of (litter-bearing) mammals, that there will be found one corpus luteum per embryo. This has been assumed to be true in the human being, and probably is true
in hormonally-induced multiple pregnancy. However, there *are* other possibilites,
and reasons for their consideration.

The closest thing to a *critical* examination of this question in the human of which we are aware resides in a paper published in 1936 by the now-deceased anatomists Wieman and Weichert. Our efforts to recover their specimen for more detailed immunological examination have so far failed. It consisted of the uterus and ovaries of a 25-year-old gunshot victim pregnant with twins. The twins were, with a probability at least in excess of 90%, dizygotic. There was only one corpus luteum.

Every ovulation has potentially four cellular-level products. The first polar body is diploid, with a set of chromosomes which do not match the set remaining in the secondary oocyte. This first polar body may divide. The secondary oocyte in the mammalian species examined to date divides shortly after sperm penetration, to form the zygote and the second polar body. There remain, then, either one or three potential "extra" haploid gametes.

One of the potential haploid daughters of the first polar body might be large enough to develop if fertilized. The same is true for the second polar body. This would require, as far as we know, only an unusually symmetrical cell division. Polar body abstriction is a sufficiently complex process (including among other elements a 90° rotation of the spindle in the cytoplasm [Austin, 1951]) to be reasonably imagined as subject to large changes in outcome from simple malfunctions. It seems at least as feasible to "lose a little bit of control" over this process as to do the same over the number of ovulations.

Twinning via fertilization of a daughter cell of the first polar body can hardly be genetically distinguished from the results of double ovulation. Counting enough corpora lutea could yield that distinction. Only when ovaries must be removed during or very shortly after dizygotic twin pregnancies will this be ethical and practical.

Second-polar-body twins, however, may be genetically detectable. Provided we can assume Hardy-Weinberg equilibrium, it is possible to test whether or not this type of twins exists, and to estimate its prevalence, from polymorphic marker data on the twins. This will be illustrated briefly, on the assumption that we have a sample of N non-MZ twin pairs with marker data on each twin (it would be better if marker data were also available on the twins' parents, but we shall assume this is not the case).

To begin with, assume we have a two-allele marker locus with all three genotypes distinguishable, gene frequencies p and $q = 1 - p$. If the twin pair is DZ in the classical sense, the marker phenotypes it displays come from the sib-pair joint distribution given by the matrix:

$$(f_{ij}) = \begin{matrix} \frac{1}{4}p^2(1+p)^2 & \frac{1}{2}p^2q(1+p) & \frac{1}{4}p^2q^2 \\ \frac{1}{2}p^2q(1+p) & pq(1+pq) & \frac{1}{2}pq^2(1+q) \\ \frac{1}{4}p^2q^2 & \frac{1}{2}pq^2(1+q) & \frac{1}{4}q^2(1+q)^2 \end{matrix} \qquad (7)$$

If, on the other hand, the twin pair is dispermic monovular, the marker pheno-types it displays come from the following joint distribution, which is the average of the distribution for parent-offspring and that for MZ twin pairs:

$$(g_{ij}) = \begin{array}{ccc} \frac{1}{2}p^2(1+p) & \frac{1}{2}p^2q & 0 \\[2mm] \frac{1}{2}p^2q & \frac{3}{2}pq & \frac{1}{2}pq^2 \\[2mm] 0 & \frac{1}{2}pq^2 & \frac{1}{2}q^2(1+q) \end{array} \qquad (8)$$

Suppose now that our sample is a random one from a population in which α of the twins are dispermic monovular, and $(1 - \alpha)$ are truly DZ. If we observe n_{ij} twin pairs in the (ij)-th cell, ie, with phenotypes i and j, the likelihood of the sample, L, is proportional to

$$\prod_{ij} [\alpha g_{ij} + (1 - \alpha)f_{ij}]^{n_{ij}},$$

and the information on (reciprocal of the variance of) the maximum likelihood estimate of α is

$$I_\alpha = -E(\frac{d^2 \ln L}{d\alpha}) = N\Sigma \frac{(g_{ij} - f_{ij})^2}{\alpha g_{ij} + (1 - \alpha)f_{ij}}$$

The lower six curves of Figure 1 show this quantity, divided by N, plotted against p for $\alpha = 0(0.1)-0.5$. Using usual asymptotic theory, we would reject the null hypothesis that $\alpha = 0$, at the 5% significance level, if the maximum likelihood estimate divided by its standard error is greater than 1.65. The power of this test is thus $\Phi[\alpha/\sigma_\alpha - 1.65]$, where Φ is the cumulative standardized normal distribution and $\sigma_\alpha = I_\alpha^{-1/2}$ is a function of the sample size N. Using the values given in Figure 1, we can calculate the power for any sample size and for various values of α; in Figure 2 the power has been plotted against N for $\alpha = 0.1(0.1)-0.5$, assuming p = 1/2, ie, the gene frequency that gives maximal power. It is clear that it would be relatively easy to detect an α value as large as 0.5 with a moderate sample size, but very difficult, using this test, to detect an α as small as 0.1.

The method that has just been outlined can easily be modified to allow for dominance (which decreases the power), or for multiple alleles (which increases the power). It is also possible to allow for the use of marker data on multiple independent loci, the joint distributions then being given by the Kronecker products of matrices such as (7) and (8). The upper six curves of Figure 1 show the information that results when marker data on four independent loci are

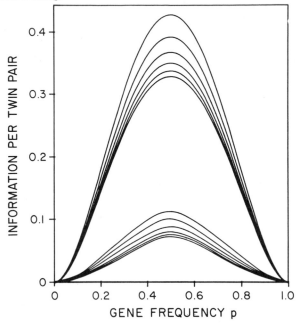

Fig. 1. Information per twin pair, I/N, as a function of marker gene frequency. The lower six curves are for one marker locus, the upper six curves are for four independent marker loci each with the same gene frequencies; the six curves correspond to the cases of (from bottom to top) $\alpha = 0$, 0.1, 0.2, 0.3, 0.4, and 0.5.

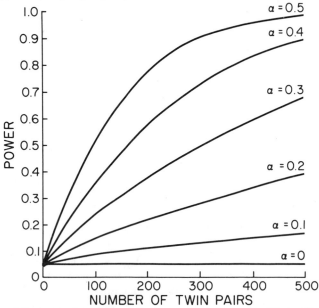

Fig. 2. Power of the test to detect dispermic monovular twins, at the 5% significance level, using a single two-allele marker locus with gene frequency 0.5.

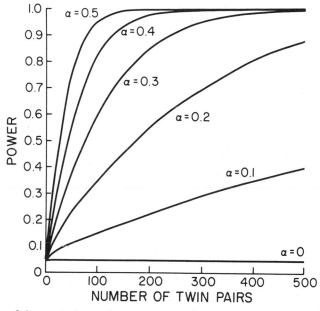

Fig. 3. Power of the test to detect dispermic monovular twins, at the 5% significance level, using four independent two-allele marker loci with gene frequency 0.5.

available, the gene frequency p being the same for all four loci, and at each two-allele locus there is no dominance; and Figure 3 gives the power calculated from these results, again for $p = 1/2$. Comparing Figure 3 with Figure 2, it is obvious that the power increases enormously as the number of marker loci increases.

To this point we have assumed that dispermic monovular twins, if they exist, will on an average be more alike genetically than ordinary sib pairs because of identity of the maternal genetic combination. However, this identity might not hold for second-polar-body twins in the presence of recombination. The sister chromatids of the primary oocyte may recombine, independently, with non-sister chromatids. They will retain identity at a given locus in the secondary oocyte only when both or neither have experienced an odd number of exchanges between that marker locus and the centromere, ie, with probability $\theta^2 + (-\theta)^2$, where θ is the probability of an odd number of crossovers between the marker and the centromere. They will be nonidentical with the complementary probability $2\theta(1 - \theta)$, and in that case the joint distribution of the marker phenotypes is the average of that for parent-offspring and that for random pairs from the population, ie, for a two-allele marker locus:

$$(h_{ij}) = \begin{matrix} \frac{1}{2}p^3(1 + p) & \frac{1}{2}p^2q(1 + 2p) & \frac{1}{2}p^2q^2 \\ \frac{1}{2}p^2q(1 + 2p) & \frac{1}{2}pq(1 + 4pq) & \frac{1}{2}pq^2(1 + 2q) \\ \frac{1}{2}p^2q^2 & \frac{1}{2}pq^2(1 + 2q) & \frac{1}{2}q^3(1 + q) \end{matrix}$$

Thus, allowing for this recombination, the likelihood of the sample is proportional to

$$\prod_{ij} \left\{ [1-\alpha] \, f_{ij} + \alpha \, [\theta^2 + (1-\theta)^2] \, g_{ij} + 2\alpha\theta \, [1-\theta] \, h_{ij} \right\}^{n_{ij}},$$

from which we can obtain maximum likelihood estimates of both α and θ provided $\alpha \neq 0$ and $\theta \neq 1/2$ [when $\theta = 1/2$, the likelihood does not depend upon α, since $f_{ij} = (g_{ij} + h_{ij})/2$]. In view of the number of twins that have already been typed for a battery of marker systems, it might well be worthwhile pooling all the available data together to determine whether or not dispermic monovular twins exist to any appreciable extent. If they do, this will tend to make Eqs (2) and (6) underestimates of σ_g^2.

In summary, the twin method is based on many assumptions, some discredited, some untested, and some untestable. In view of this, we have serious reservations about the use of the twin method by itself to estimate genetic variance or heritability. Only with the greatest of circumspection may the results of genetic twin studies ever be considered to represent the general population, or be appropriately melded with data from pairs of singleton relatives in tests of genetic models. Rao et al [1976] consider "perhaps it is time to suggest that, for its contribution to biometric genetics, twin research might profitably be left to twins." We do not mean to argue that twin research is of little use, but rather that twin research should have entirely *different* and more promising uses. There is no question that the differences within pairs of MZ twins indicate extranuclear influences, and that twins have undergone a unique kind of embryological development. It is time we capitalized on these aspects of twins, rather than on their use to estimate heritability.

ACKNOWLEDGMENTS

This investigation was supported by a US Public Health Service Research Scientist Award (MH31732) from the National Institute of Mental Health, and a training grant (GM00006) and research grant (GM16697) from the National Institute of General Medical Sciences.

REFERENCES

Austin CR (1951): Observations on the penetration of the sperm into the mammalian egg. Aust J Sci Res 4:581–596.

Boklage CE (1977a): Schizophrenia, brain asymmetry development and twinning: A cellular relationship with etiological and possibly prognostic implications. Biol Psychiatry 12(1): 19–35.

Boklage CE (1977b): Some questions about schizophrenia in twins. Discussion paper prepared for the Rochester Second International Conference on Schizophrenia.

Bulmer MG (1970): "The Biology of Twinning in Man." Oxford: Clarendon Press.

Christian JC, Kang KW, Norton JA Jr (1974): Choice of an estimate of genetic variance from twin data. Am J Hum Genet 26:154–161.

Christian JC, Kang KW, Norton JA Jr (1977): Comparison of within-pair and among-component estimates of genetic variance from twin data. Letter to the Editor. Am J Hum Genet 29:208–210.

Cockerham CC (1954): An extension of the concept of partitioning hereditary variance for analysis of covariance among relatives when epistasis is present. Genetics 39:859–882.

Corey LA, Kang KW, Christian JC, Norton JA Jr, Harris RE, Nance WE (1976): Effects of chorion type on variation in cord blood cholesterol of monozygotic twins. Am J Hum Genet 28:433–441.

Corner GW (1955): The observed embryology of human single-ovum twins and other multiple births. Am J Obstet Gynecol 70:935–951.

Gaines RE, Elston RC (1969): On the probability that a twin pair is monozygotic. Am J Hum Genet 21:457–465.

Haseman JK, Elston RC (1970): The estimation of genetic variance from twin data. Behav Genet 1:11–19.

Jinks JL, Fulker DW (1970): Comparison of the biometrical, genetical, MAVA, and classical approaches to the analysis of human behavior. Psychol Bull 73:311–349.

Li CC (1976): "First Course in Population Genetics." Pacific Grove, California: The Boxwood Press.

Morton NE (1974): Analysis of family resemblance. I. Introduction. Am J Hum Genet 26:318–330.

Nance WE (1976): Note on the analysis of twin data. Letter to the Editor. Am J Hum Genet 28:297–298.

Rao DC, Morton NE, Yee S (1976): Resolution of cultural and biological inheritance by path analysis. Am J Hum Genet 28:228–242.

Strong SJ, Corney G (1967): "The Placenta in Twin Pregnancy." Oxford: Pergamon Press.

Taubman P (1976): The determinants of earnings: Genetics, family, and other environments; a study of white male twins. Am Econ Rev 66:858–870.

Weiman HL, Weichert CK (1936): Anat Rec 65:201.

The Monozygotic Half-Sib Model: A Tool for Epidemiologic Research

Linda A Corey and Walter E Nance

Over the years, numerous methodologies have been developed to examine the origins of observed variation in quantitative traits in man. Most of these approaches, however, have been faced either with the usual biases associated with the use of abnormal relationships, such as twins reared apart or adopted children, or with the need to collect vast bodies of data in order to remove effects of confounding in parameter estimates. Although genetic and environmental components of variance have been estimated in numerous studies of quantitative traits in man, the experimental designs of previous studies permitted neither an unambiguous assessment of the relative importance of each in the expression of the trait nor a determination of the contribution of maternal effects, a factor which might strongly influence the expression of such traits.

A new approach which utilizes the children of identical twins provides a means of assessing genetic and environmental influences on quantitative traits [Nance, 1976; Nance and Corey, 1976] as well as for resolving much of the controversy surrounding the etiology of certain multifactorial traits [Corey et al, in press]. By taking advantage of the unique relationship between identical twins but not focusing on the twins themselves, this model circumvents many of the problems associated with classical twin and nuclear family studies. As shown in Figure 1, the children of each member of an identical twin pair are related to each other as half-siblings. Each half-sib family contains individuals who have all of their genes, one-half of their genes, one-quarter of their genes, and none of their genes in common. The different genetic relationships present in half-sib families provide a means by which estimates of genetic and environmental components can be obtained. Maternal effects can be detected through a comparison of the manner in which observed variation is partitioned among and within families of male and female identical twins.

Twin Research: Psychology and Methodology, pages 201–209

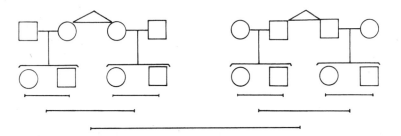

Fig 1. Structure of monozygotic half-sib data

The nested analyses of variance used to examine variation in half-sib families are shown in Table I. The mean squares obtained from these analyses, together with the mean squares obtained from analyses of variance among and within twin pairs and the mean cross products obtained from analyses of covariance between different classes of relatives, when set equal to their respective expectations provide estimates of genetic, maternal, and environmental components through an iterative weighted least-squares procedure. The rationale and methodology used to obtain these estimates have been discussed in detail by Nance and Corey [1976].

Although this model permits the detection of maternal effects, it does not separate cytoplasmic effects from effects of prenatal environment or from genetically determined maternal effects. To distinguish among those effects, the model must be extended to include the grandchildren of identical twins. As shown in Figure 2, the grandchildren of each member of an identical twin pair are related to each other as 1½ cousins.

The variation observed in grandchildren of identical twins can be partitioned by a nested analysis of variance similar to that used to partition variation in the children of identical twins. The analysis involves two levels of nesting as shown in Table II. Because there are usually unequal numbers of grandchildren in each sibship, components estimated by the nested analysis are weighted, as shown in the table.

Based upon the sexes of the twin grandparents, their children, and their grandchildren, there are 20 distinct types of 1½ cousinships as shown in Figure 3. Analysis of characters within these different relationships, in conjunction with the previously described half-sib analysis, provides a powerful and definitive methodological tool for the examination of epidemiological variables. In particular, it permits a clear resolution of nuclear, cytoplasmic, and environmental maternal effects if the following assumptions are valid: 1) The female parent is the sole contributor of cytoplasmic DNA to the zygote, 2) the nuclear genotype of the maternal parent has no permanent effect on the constitution of cytoplasmic DNA of germ cells transmitted from generation to generation, and 3) cytoplasmic traits

TABLE I. Analysis of Variance of Half-Sib Data

Source of variation	Degree of freedom	Mean square	Expected mean square
Among half-sibships	$N - 1$	MSA	$\sigma_W^2 + b_2\sigma_B^2 + a\sigma_A^2$
Between sibships within half-sibships	N	MSB	$\sigma_W^2 + b_1\sigma_B^2$
Within sibships	$\Sigma(n_{i1} + n_{i2}) - 2N$	MSW	σ_W^2
Total	$\Sigma(n_{i1} + n_{i2}) - 1$	MST	

$$b_1 = \frac{\Sigma(n_{i1} + n_{i2}) - [\Sigma(n_{i1}^2 + n_{i2}^2)/(n_{i1} + n_{i2})]}{N}$$

$$b_2 = \frac{\Sigma(n_{i1}^2 + n_{i2}^2)/(n_{i1} + n_{i2}) - [\Sigma(n_{i1}^2 + n_{i2}^2)/\Sigma(n_{i1} + n_{i2})]}{N - 1}$$

$$a = \frac{\Sigma(n_{i1} + n_{i2}) - [(n_{i1} + n_{i2})^2/\Sigma(n_{i1} + n_{i2})]}{N - 1}$$

TABLE II. Analysis of Variance for Data on the Grandchildren of Identical Twins*

Source of variation	Degrees of Freedom	Mean Square	Expected mean square
Among 1½ cousinships	$N-1$	MSAC	$\sigma^2_W + s_3\sigma^2_{BS} + c_2\sigma^2_{BC} + a\sigma^2_A$
Between first cousinships nested within 1½ cousinships	N	MSBC	$\sigma^2_W + s_2\sigma^2_{BS} + c_1\sigma^2_{BC}$
Between full sibships nested within first cousinships	$2N$	MSBS	$\sigma^2_W + s_1\sigma^2_{BS}$
Within full sibships	$\sum_i(n_{ij1} + n_{ij2})-4N$	MSW	σ^2_W

$$s_1 = \frac{\sum\sum_{ij}(n_{ij1} + n_{ij2})-[\sum\sum_{ij}(n_{ij1}^2 + n_{ij2}^2)/n_{ij.}]}{2N}$$

$$s_2 = \frac{[\sum\sum_{ij}(n_{ij1}^2 + n_{ij2}^2)/n_{ij.}]-[\sum\sum_{ij}(n_{ij1}^2 + n_{ij2}^2)/n_{i..}]}{N}$$

$$s_3 = \frac{[\sum\sum_{ij}(n_{ij1}^2 + n_{ij2}^2)/N]-[\sum\sum_{ij}(n_{ij1}^2 + n_{ij2}^2)/\sum\sum_{ij}(n_{ij1} + n_{ij2})]}{N-1}$$

$$c_1 = \frac{[\sum\sum_{ij}(n_{ij1} + n_{ij2})^2/n_{ij.}]-[\sum\sum_{ij}(n_{ij1} + n_{ij2})^2/n_{i..}]}{N}$$

$$c_2 = \frac{[\sum\sum_{ij}(n_{ij1} + n_{ij2})^2/n_{i..}]-[(\sum\sum_{ij}(n_{ij1} + n_{ij2}))^2/\sum\sum_{ij}(n_{ij1} + n_{ij2})]}{N-1}$$

$$a = \frac{\sum\sum_{ij}(n_{ij1} + n_{ij2})-[\sum_i(\sum_j(n_{ij1} + n_{ij2}))^2/\sum\sum_{ij}(n_{ij1} + n_{ij2})]}{N-1}$$

*Model given assumes a symmetrical design with two fertile offspring for each twin but unequal sibship size among the grandchildren. N = number of 1½ cousinships; n = number of grandchildren in each sibship.

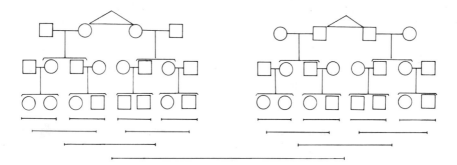

Fig 2. Structure of data of grandchildren of identical twins.

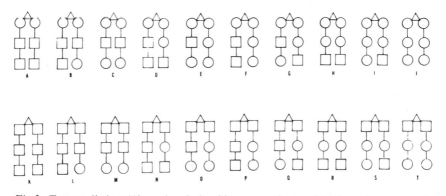

Fig 3. Twenty distinct 1½ cousin relationships among the grandchildren of monozygotic twins.

remain stable and do not segregate from one generation to the next. For example, all matrilineal grandchildren (1½ cousins) of a female identical twin pair should share identical cytoplasmic DNA, whereas the patrilineal grandchildren (1½ cousins) of a female identical twin pair would have no cytoplasmic DNA in common (Fig 2). Therefore, if the expression of a given trait were influenced by the cytoplasm, one would expect to see less variation between matrilineal grandchildren of a female twin than between matrilineal grandchildren of male twins or patrilineal grandchildren of either male twins or female twins. On the other hand, if the expression of a trait were conditioned by genetically determined maternal effects, one would expect to see less variation between matrilineal grandchildren of either male or female twin pairs than between patrilineal grandchildren. To the degree that the extended-twin-family model (hereafter called twin-kinship model) permits a more exact partitioning of observed variation into maternal and environmental sources, comparisons of variation among and within families will permit a clearer resolution of genetic components of variance than that provided by the half-sib model. Data on discontinuous traits such as birth defects can be approached in an analogous manner. However, instead of comparing the variation in the trait among and within matrilineal and patrilineal grandchildren of male and female identical twins, one would compare frequencies of the trait's expression for each class of relatives. Comparisons of the incidence of specific birth defects, for example, in patrilineal and matrilineal grandchildren of male and female identical twins will permit the detection of both cytoplasmic and maternal influences and, in addition, will allow their formal resolution from effects of X-linked genes. The structure of three selected matrilineal and patrilineal 1½ cousinships is given in Figure 4. The genetic, cytoplasmic, maternal, and environmental expectations for the three selected nested analyses of variance of grandchildren (associated with these particular family types) are given in Figure 5. The between full sibships within first cousinship partition for patrilineal grandchildren of male identical twins contains variation resulting from both cytoplasmic and genetically determined maternal effects; in this case, all of the similarities between grandchildren attributable to maternal effects are determined by genetically unrelated mothers. On the other hand, the variation resulting from cytoplasmic effects seen in maternal grandchildren of male identical twins appears in the between first cousinship within 1½ cousinship partition of variance (II-BC), while fractions of the genetically determined maternal effect are contained in the among 1½ cousinship, between first cousinship nested within 1½

Patrilineal grandchildren of male identical twins

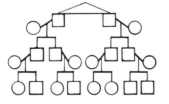

Matrilineal grandchildren of male identical twins

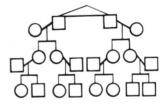

Matrilineal grandchildren of female identical twins

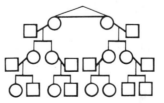

Fig 4. Structure of three selected matrilineal and patrilineal 1½ cousinships.

cousinships, and between full sibships nested within first cousinships partitions of variance. In these families, there is no variance in cytoplasmic effects with cousinships since they arise from women who were full sisters. Finally, variation arising from cytoplasmic effects occurs in the among 1½ cousinship partition of variance for matrilineal grandchildren of female identical twins. There should be no variation in cytoplasmic effects within the entire kinship in this situation. Variation resulting from genetically determined maternal effects, as is true of matrilineal grandchildren of male identical twins, should be estimated in part by the among 1½ cousinships, in part by the between first cousinships nested within 1½ cousinships, and in part by the between full sibships nested within first cousinships partitions of variance. As shown in Figure 5 the distribution of genetically determined maternal effects depends upon the degree to which the mothers of the grandchildren are related. By equating the expectation for each partition of variance or covariance to its corresponding observed mean square or mean cross product and solving these equations simultaneously, direct estimates of genetically determined maternal and cytoplasmic components of variance as well as direct genetic (V_A, V_D, etc) and environmental components can be obtained. The model has also been extended to include four sources of environmental variance: V_{EC}, or the variation associated with 1½ cousinships; V_{EF}, or the variation associated with full cousinships; V_{ES}, or the variation associated with full sibships; and V_{EW_D}, or the variation within full sibships. This categorization will reveal environmental variance associated with particular familial relationships. In addition, the twin-kinship model also removes any biases that might be introduced by the inclusion of multigenerational comparisons since the equations for analysis of the grandchildren are sufficient to confine analysis to individuals of the same generation, thus eliminating the need to include parent-offspring regressions in the overall analysis.

Eaves [1972] has shown that, when a quantitative genetic analysis is confined to the relationships in which the parameters to be estimated are largely confounded, vast amounts of data are required to detect significant effects. The power of the methodology presented herein lies in the fact that the relationships that exist within this family structure provide multiple equations and contrasts in which additive, dominance, maternal, and environmental effects are not confounded. As is true of classical twin studies, half-sib and twin-kinship studies may be complicated by serious ascertainment biases. Although many of the possible biases associated with dizygotic twin studies, ie, effects of maternal age, parity, race, etc, are circumvented by examining monozygotic twins and their progeny, some bias from socioeconomic status, educational level, or the existence of close personal relationships between adult twins may be introduced when twin pairs taking part in the study are self-selected. Therefore, the safest and most effective approach is to use a population-based sample, where the twin pairs and their families might be located through a search of birth records, for example. A twin

PARTITION	VARIANCE COMPONENT	V_A	V_D	V_{AA}	V_{DD}	V_{AD}	V_{AM}	V_{DM}	V_C	V_{EC}	V_{EF}	V_{ES}	V_{EW}
1. PATRILINEAL GRANDCHILDREN OF MALE IDENTICAL TWINS													
Among 1½ Cousinships	σ^2_A	1/16	0	1/256	0	0	0	0	0	1	0	0	0
Between First Cousins/ 1½ Cousinships	σ^2_{BC}	1/16	0	3/256	0	0	0	0	0	0	1	0	0
Between Full Sibs/ First Cousinships	σ^2_{BS}	3/8	1/4	15/64	1/16	1/8	1	1	1	0	0	1	0
Within Full Sibships	σ^2_W	1/2	3/4	3/4	15/16	7/8	0	0	0	0	0	0	1
2. MATRILINEAL GRANDCHILDREN OF MALE IDENTICAL TWINS													
Among 1½ Cousinships	σ^2_A	1/16	0	1/256	0	0	1/4	0	0	1	0	0	0
Between First Cousins/ 1½ Cousinships	σ^2_{BC}	1/16	0	3/256	0	0	1/4	1/4	1	0	1	0	0
Between Full Sibs/ First Cousinships	σ^2_{BS}	3/8	1/4	15/64	1/16	1/8	1/2	3/4	0	0	0	1	0
Within Full Sibships	σ^2_W	1/2	3/4	3/4	15/16	7/8	0	0	0	0	0	0	1
3. MATRILINEAL GRANDCHILDREN OF FEMALE IDENTICAL TWINS													
Among 1½ Cousinships	σ^2_A	1/16	0	1/256	0	0	1/4	0	1	1	0	0	0
Between First Cousins/ 1½ Cousinships	σ^2_{BC}	1/16	0	3/256	0	0	1/4	1/4	0	0	1	0	0
Between Full Sibs/ First Cousinships	σ^2_{BS}	3/8	1/4	15/64	1/16	1/8	1/2	3/4	0	0	0	1	0
Within Full Sibships	σ^2_W	1/2	3/4	3/4	15/16	7/8	0	0	0	0	0	0	1

Fig 5. Expectations for nested analyses of selected offspring of male and female MZ twins.

panel of this type has the added advantage that epidemiological variables in the population as a whole can be monitored on a yearly basis through an examination of children born to identical twins. Preliminary data from a pilot study to locate children with congenital malformations born to identical twins reveal that, of the approximately 75,000 births per year in Virginia alone, there are approximately 325 children born to a parent who is an identical twin. A panel of this type, including individuals from several states, would yield a pool of information more than adequate for relevant estimates of genetic and environmental sources of variation as well as for monitoring characteristics.

SUMMARY

The half-sib and twin-kinship models provide an important tool for the examination of variation in quantitative traits in man and for the investigation of the etiology of multifactorial traits. This methodology also permits partitioning of previously confounded types of maternal effects, ie, cytoplasmic, environmental, and genetic, and consequently, examination of previously unrecognized sources of variation in quantitative traits.

ACKNOWLEDGMENTS

This is paper No. 49 from the Department of Human Genetics of the Medical College of Virginia and was supported in part by NIH grant 1 P01HD10291.

REFERENCES

Corey LA, Nance WE, Berg K (in press): A new tool in birth defect research: The MZ half-sib model and its extension to grandchildren of identical twins. In Summitt R (ed): "Birth Defects." New York: Alan R. Liss.

Eaves LJ (1972): Computer simulation of sample size and experimental design in human psychogenetics. Psychol Bull 77:144–152.

Nance WE (1976): Genetic studies of the offspring of identical twins. Acta Genet Med Gemellol (Roma) 25:103–113.

Nance WE, Corey LA (1976): Genetic models for the analysis of data from families of identical twins. Genetics 83:811–826

Familial Resemblance in Patterns of Growth in Stature

R Darrell Bock

It is well known that measures of stature show considerable resemblance within families. Estimates of the heritability coefficient for mature stature fall in the range 0.7 to 0.8, comparable to those for resemblance of intellectual ability [Osborne and De George, 1959]. It is also believed that the pattern of growth in stature exhibits familial similarity, but difficulties in characterizing the rather complex shape of the human growth curve for stature have hindered quantitative estimation of heritability of pattern. Vandenberg and Falkner [1965] made an attempt along these lines using an orthogonal polynomial resolution of a segment of the growth curve of twins. In the age range from birth to 5 years, they found greater concordance between identical twins than between fraternals only for the quadratic component of growth (ie, for rate of deceleration of growth during early childhood). Other components showed no evidence of heritability. Although this method of characterizing growth pattern is straightforward, it does not readily generalize to wider age spans. The difficulty is that the orthogonal polynomials do not give a good account of larger segments of the growth curve, especially if the adolescent age range is included.

In an attempt to find a better functional representation of human growth in stature, Bock et al [1973] proposed the use of a compound curve consisting of two additive logistic components — one characterizing prepubertal growth, and the other, the adolescent growth spurt. This curve proved easy to fit by unweighted nonlinear least squares, and gave an approximate description of growth, in terms of six interpretable parameters, from 1 year to maturity. But the fit of this curve was not as close as might be desired, especially in the age range just prior to adolescence. Bock and Thissen [1976] ultimately came to the conclusion that the rapid deceleration of growth in early childhood could not be represented accurately by a single logistic component. They therefore proposed that prepubertal

Twin Research: Psychology and Methodology, pages 211–216

growth in stature be represented by the sum of two logistic components in the proportions p and $1 - p$. This proposal was similar in many respects to those advanced earlier by Robertson [1908] and Burt [1937] but never implemented because of computational difficulties. With the aid of the Fletcher-Powell minimization procedure, however, Bock and Thissen [1976] were able to fit the triple-logistic curve by unweighted nonlinear least squares. This function gave an extraordinarily good fit to growth in stature in the range from 1 year to maturity. Almost to the limit of the measurement error (about 0.5 cm root mean square), the triple-logistic curve expresses in terms of nine parameters every detail of individual growth in stature. It presents the possibility of characterizing familial resemblance in pattern of growth in terms of heritability coefficients for these parameters. Or, alternatively, it may be used to "graduate" the growth curve so that derivatives of the curve can be accurately estimated and used descriptively.

This approach is applied in the present paper to an examination of patterns of growth in stature in two sets of triplets whose measures of height from near birth to maturity are part of the first generation Fels longitudinal growth study. In each set, two sibs are identical, and the other is fraternal. These cases of multiple birth were recruited from a "twin" club active in Springfield, Ohio, during the 1930s. I am indebted to Dr Alex Roche of Fels Institute for supplying the data for these subjects, all of whom grew to maturity without notable medical or developmental problems. Surprisingly, these interesting cases, enrolled in the Fels growth-study in the 1930s, have never been described in the literature.

Figure 1 shows the fitted triple-logistic growth curves for the set of male triplets. The identical sibs are represented by solid lines, and the fraternal by a broken line. Figure 2 shows curves for a similar set of female triplets. The curves of the identical sibs are by no means coincident and demonstrate the considerable extent to which cumulative nonheritable effects can produce individual differences in the timing of growth, although not in final stature. Nevertheless, the curves of the identical sibs are clearly more similar to each other than to that of the fraternal sibs. Were the zygosities of the triplets not known (from serology in this case), the growth curves would accurately identify the identical sibs. The question of present interest is: How is this similarity reflected in the fitted parameters or descriptive features of the triple-logistic growth curves?

The function proposed by Bock and Thissen is as follows:

$$Y = A1 \left\{ \frac{1-p}{1 + \exp\left[-B1\left(t - C1\right)\right]} + \frac{p}{1 + \exp\left[-B2\left(t - C2\right)\right]} \right\} + A3 \frac{1}{1 + \exp\left[-B3(t - C3)\right]} ,$$

where $A1$ is the total contribution of the prepubertal component to mature stature (cm); $B1$ is the maximum velocity (logits/year) of the first prepubertal component; $C1$ is the age (years) at maximum velocity of the first prepubertal

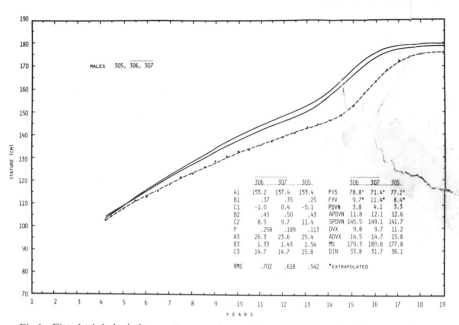

MALES 305, 306, 307

	306	307	305		306	307	305
A1	153.2	157.4	153.4	FYS	78.8*	71.4*	77.2*
B1	.37	.35	.25	FYV	9.7*	11.4*	8.4*
C1	-1.0	0.4	-0.1	PDVN	3.8	4.1	3.3
B2	.45	.50	.43	APDVN	11.8	12.1	12.6
C2	8.5	9.7	11.4	SPDVN	145.5	149.1	141.7
P	.258	.189	.113	DVX	9.8	9.7	11.2
A3	26.3	23.6	25.4	ADVX	14.5	14.7	15.8
B3	1.33	1.43	1.54	MS	179.3	180.8	177.8
C3	14.7	14.7	15.8	DIN	33.8	31.7	36.1
RMS	.702	.618	.542	*EXTRAPOLATED			

Fig 1. Fitted triple-logistic growth curves for a set of male triplets, based on annual and semiannual measures of stature made at Fels Institute.

component; $B2$ is the maximum velocity (logits/year) of the second prepubertal component; $C2$ is the age (years) at the maximum velocity of the second prepubertal component; p is the proportion of the prepubertal contribution to stature attributable to the second component; $A3$ is the contribution of the adolescent component to mature stature (cm); $B3$ is the maximum velocity (logits/year) of the adolescent component; and $C3$ is the age (years) at maximum velocity of the adolescent component.

In addition to characterizing the curves by the parameters of their latent components, we may also compute from the fitted functions certain descriptive features of the manifest curves. The following quantities are proposed for this purpose: 1) first year stature (FYS), 2) first year velocity (FYV), 3) Preadolescent velocity minimum (PDVN), 4) stature at preadolescent velocity minimum (SPVDN), 5) age at preadolescent velocity minimum (APDVN), 6) adolescent velocity maximum (DVX), 7) age at adolescent velocity maximum (ADVX), 8) mature stature (MS), and 9) adolescent increment to stature (DIN).

Any of these characterizations of the growth curves are, of course, valid only to the extent that the fitted functions accurately reflect the data. Some indication of the goodness of fit of the triple-logistic function is seen in the plotted curve for the nonidentical subject in Figure 1, which includes the data points

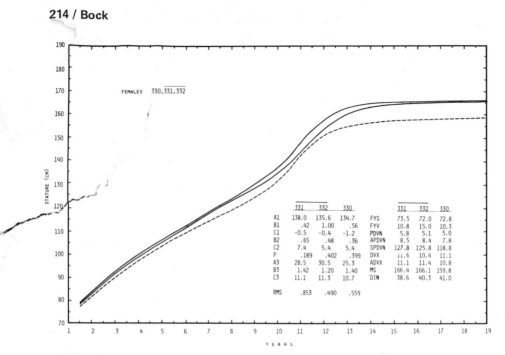

		331	332	330		331	332	330
	A1	138.0	135.6	134.7	FYS	73.5	72.0	72.8
	B1	.42	1.00	.56	FYV	10.8	15.0	10.3
	C1	-0.5	-0.4	-1.2	PDVN	5.8	5.1	5.0
	B2	.65	.48	.36	APDVN	8.5	8.4	7.8
	C2	7.4	5.4	5.4	SPDVN	127.8	125.8	118.8
	P	.189	.402	.399	DVX	11.6	10.4	11.1
	A3	28.5	30.5	25.3	ADVX	11.1	11.4	10.8
	B3	1.42	1.20	1.40	MS	166.4	166.1	159.8
	C3	11.1	11.3	10.7	DIN	38.6	40.3	41.0
	RMS	.853	.490	.559				

Fig 2. Fitted triple-logistic growth curves for a set of female triplets, based on annual and semiannual measures of stature made at Fels Institute.

as well as the theoretical curve. The width of each point is approximately two standard errors of measurement (± 0.5 cm) as estimated for the Fels procedure from repeated annual measurements of mature stature. It is apparent that only a few of the observed measurements differ from the fitted curve by more than one standard error.

More formally, the root mean square residuals, shown at the lower right of each figure, are all comparable to the root mean square measurement error.

The only case in the present data for which the fit might be questioned is number 331. The rather large root mean square of 0.853 cm for this subject proves to have resulted largely from a discrepant observation at 21 years of age. Inasmuch as the final three annual measurements at 20, 21, and 22 years of age were 166.4, 169.0 and 166.9 cm, a clerical error must be suspected.

If the accuracy of the triple-logistic functions in representing the actual growth of these subjects can be accepted, we should expect that the greater similarity of the identical sibs that is apparent visually would be conveyed in some way in the parameters of the functions, or in the descriptive features. Those quantities that reflect similarity will show a smaller difference between the identical sibs than between the identical sibs and the fraternal sibs.

Applying this criterion to the parameter estimates in Figure 1, we see that only C2, age at the velocity maximum of the second prepubertal component, and C3, age at the velocity maximum of the adolescent component, are indicative of similarity of the identical male sibs.

For the female triplets in Figure 2, C3, A3 (the adolescent contribution to mature stature), and C1 (the age at the first prepubertal velocity maximum) are indicative, but C2 is not. In terms of parameters, only the age location of the adolescent growth spurt is a consistent indicator of the similarity of growth patterns of the identical sibs.

Turning to the descriptive features of the curves, we find more indication of similarities. For the male triplets, all of the descriptive features satisfy the criterion, except first year stature and first year velocity. In these data, however, the observations do not start until 4 years of age, and the first year figures are extrapolations. The value for the first year stature extrapolated for subject 307 is not very plausible, however, and is probably an extrapolation error. Typically, growth curves of same-sex siblings are quite similar around 1 year of age, so we might not expect the first year figures to be useful for distinguishing identical twins from fraternal twins.

In the girls' data, the considerable divergence in the identical sibs' timing of the adolescent growth spurt makes the PDVN, DVX, and ADVX features useless as indicators, but APDVN and SPDVN (the age and stature at the preadolescent velocity minimum) are useful, as is MS (mature stature). Note that this difference in stature was present before adolescence and was not the result of the amount of adolescent growth.

For the girls as for the boys, the first year figures do not distinguish the identical from the fraternal sibs.

The inspection of these data for growth in stature of triplets, which provide a rare opportunity to compare identical and fraternal sibs of the same age in the same family environment, leave the general impression that the heritable aspect of growth pattern, as opposed to mere difference in mature stature, involves primarily the appearance of the adolescent growth spurt. Only this component of growth shows enough variability in its effect on pattern to be useful as an indicator of heritable effects in development of stature. Although the adolescent contribution can be characterized by the third component of the triple-logistic function, it may also be characterized in the manifest growth curve by the minimum of the preadolescent velocity, which has been used (for example, by Tanner et al. [1976]) to mark the age of onset of adolescence — by the adolescent maximum velocity, which measures the steepness of the spurt, by the age of the maximum, which best locates the adolescent event, and by the contribution of adolescent growth to mature stature. The triple-logistic curve provides an accurate method of determining these quantities in data for individual growth in stature.

REFERENCES

Bock RD, Thissen DM (1976): Fitting multi-component models for growth in stature. In "Proceedings of the Ninth International Biometrics Conference." Volume 1, pp 431–432.

Bock RD, Wainer H, Petersen A, Thissen D, Murray J, Roche A (1973): A parameterization for individual human growth curves. Hum Biol 45:63–80.

Burt C (1937): "The Backward Child." New York: Appleton-Century-Crofts.

Osborne RH, De George FV (1959): "Genetic Basis of Morphological Variation." Cambridge, Mass: Harvard University Press.

Robertson TB (1908): On the normal rate of growth of an individual and its biochemical significance. Arch Entwickl Mechan Organism 25:581–614.

Tanner JM, Whitehouse RH, Marubini E, Resele IF (1976): The adolescent growth spurt of boys and girls of the Harpenden Growth Study. Ann Hum Biol 3:109–126.

Vandenberg SG, Falkner F (1965): Hereditary factors in growth: Twin concordances on growth curves. Hum Biol 37:357–365.

Multivariate Extensions of a Biometrical Model of Twin Data

DW Fulker

In this paper I would like to discuss some of the problems involved in the multivariate analysis of twin data and describe a maximum likelihood approach that goes some way towards solving them.

Partitioning phenotypic covariance into genetic and environmental components for the purpose of investigating their structure was first suggested by Tukey in 1951. He made the point, novel at the time, that just as mean squares in analysis of variance could be partitioned into components, mean cross products in analysis of covariance could also be partitioned in a completely analogous fashion. Subsequently the structure of these component matrices could be explored to indicate how genetic and environmental influences caused measures to become associated.

The idea of looking at twin data in this way appears to have been first suggested by Kempthorne and Osborne in 1961, ten years later, without reference to Tukey's original discussion of the problem. However, in recognition of his contribution, and because his illustrative example involving four protein levels in single crosses of maize demonstrates the multivariate approach so well, I would like to discuss it briefly by way of introduction.

The analysis is the simplest possible, following a one-way analysis of variance, and is shown in Table I. The top part of the table shows the two 4×4 matrices of mean cross products, one between crosses (B_{ij}), the other within (W_{ij}). Subscripted matrix notation will be used wherever possible in order to emphasize the simple one-to-one or element-for-element correspondence that frequently exists between observed covariances and multivariate models. The estimate of the environmental covariance matrix, $\hat{E}_{ij}$, is given directly by W_{ij}, while the initial estimate of the genetic component $_1\hat{G}_{ij}$, is given by one-quarter of the difference between B_{ij} and W_{ij}, there being four replications.

Twin Research: Psychology and Methodology, pages 217–236

TABLE I. ANCOVA of Four Proteins in Maize [Tukey, 1951]*

	Between crosses (8 df)				z_i	Expectations	Correlations			
B_{ij}	860.4	178.9	146.3	86.2		$B_{ij} = E_{ij} + 4G_{ij}$				
		43.3	33.4	17.9		$W_{ij} = E_{ij}$				
			30.8	13.1						
				9.4						

	Within crosses (27 df)				z_i		Correlations			
W_{ij}	49.1	10.4	5.6	2.3		RE_{ij}	1.00	0.35	0.52	0.41
		6.0	0.4	0.6				1.00	0.10	0.31
			2.4	0.2					1.00	0.17
				0.6						1.00
$_1\hat{G}_{ij}$	202.8	42.1	35.2	21.0		RG_{ij}	1.00	0.97	0.94	0.99
		9.3	8.3	4.3				1.00	1.01	0.95
			7.1	3.2					1.00	0.81
				2.2						1.00
$_2\hat{G}_{ij} = z_i z_j$	202.8	43.4	35.7	20.1	14.24	RG_{ij}	1.00	1.00	1.00	1.00
		9.3	7.7	4.3	3.05			1.00	1.00	1.00
			6.3	3.6	2.51				1.00	1.00
				2.0	1.41					1.00

*Note: B_{ij}, between crosses mean cross products; W_{ij}, within crosses mean cross products; $_1\hat{G}_{ij}$, first estimate of genetic covariance matrix; $_2\hat{G}_{ij}$, second estimate of genetic covariance matrix; z_i, first principal component of G_{ij}; RE_{ij}, correlation matrix corresponding to E_{ij}; and RG_{ij}, correlation matrix corresponding to G_{ij}.

The structures of the genetic and environmental matrices are quite different, as can be seen from their corresponding correlation matrices, RG_{ij} and RE_{ij}, shown to the right of the table. The environmental correlations are quite small. Evidently, so far as the environment is concerned, the four proteins are to a large extent independently determined, their levels responding differently to particular conditions of soil and climate. The genetic covariance matrix, on the other hand, shows a very high degree of association, the correlations hardly differing from unity. In contrast to the environment, all four protein levels appear to be determined by a single, in this case, genetic system.

When all the values in a correlation matrix approach 1, its unitary structure can be expressed as a single factor or principal component. Tukey estimated the four loadings, $\hat{z}_i$, of the first principal component from his initial estimate of the genetic component matrix, $_1\hat{G}_{ij}$, forming a new estimate, $_2\hat{G}_{ij}$, as the corresponding products of these loadings, $\hat{z}_i\hat{z}_j$. This component is shown in the column at the foot of the table and accounts for over 99% of the initial estimate of genetic variance. It appears, by eye, to fit the data very well, providing a more parsimonious explanation of the genetic covariance structure and lending support to the hypothesis of a single genetic system.

This direct structural approach to the analysis of component matrices bypasses the main difficulty of the additive approach that estimates components by taking the difference between matrices of observed mean cross products. In the additive approach, variances may take impossible negative values so that correlations cannot be estimated and even when variances are positive, correlations may fall well outside the range of ± 1. Structural analysis of such matrices, which are the rule rather than the exception, may prove impossible.

However, component matrices based on principal components behave exactly like those based directly on paired observations, their latent roots all being $\geqslant 0$. Matrices conforming to this constraint are sometimes referred to as Gramian and present no problems for further structural analysis, should this be deemed necessary. The problem is, however, how many principal components are needed to account for any particular set of data adequately, and how do we estimate them?

With characteristic insight, Tukey indicated that a multivariate extension of the F ratio might be developed to establish the required rank of a component matrix. In the same year Bartlett [1951] published just such a procedure for use in discriminant analysis. This procedure was that later adopted by Bock and Vandenberg [1968] to obtain constrained estimates of the genetic covariance matrix from twin data.

Their method uses the within-pair cross product matrices for dizygotic (DZ) and monozygotic (MZ) twins, DZW_{ij} and MZW_{ij} or **DZW** and **MZW** in conventional matrix notation. The rank of the genetic covariance matrix is estimated as the number of latent roots greater than unity in the multivariate analysis of variance determinantal equation developed by Bartlett,

$$| \mathbf{DZW} - \Lambda\mathbf{MZW} | = 0,$$

where Λ is the diagonal matrix of roots. Those less than unity, which roughly correspond to negative roots in the component matrix, are set to unity to form Λ^*. This modified matrix of roots is combined with the discriminant functions, $\mathbf{X}$, to estimate the genetic covariance matrix as

$$(\mathbf{X}^{-1})'(\Lambda^* - \mathbf{I})(\mathbf{X}^{-1}).$$

The estimated matrix will be Gramian and can be subjected to further structural analysis by a variety of established procedures.

The method is very straightforward, economical in terms of computer time, and has recently been shown by Bock and Petersen [1975] to provide a constrained maximum likelihood estimate of G_{ij}. It is the only method currently available that provides an explicit solution to the multivariate problem and has been used successfully in a number of applications [Bock and Vandenberg, 1968; Eaves, 1973; Nance et al., 1974].

However, in spite of its considerable advantages, it does suffer from a number of drawbacks. Firstly, it is wasteful of data. In the case of twins, only the within-pairs information is used, that between pairs being excluded from the analysis. The evaluation of more extensive kinships would be even more wasteful, if possible at all. Secondly, the method cannot deal with more than the simplest basic twin model, as we can see if we consider the model below.

$$\begin{aligned} \mathbf{MZB}_{ij} &= \mathbf{SE}_{ij} + 2\mathbf{G}_{ij} + 2\mathbf{CE}_{ij}, \\ \mathbf{MZW}_{ij} &= \mathbf{SE}_{ij}, \\ \mathbf{DZB}_{ij} &= \mathbf{SE}_{ij} + 1\tfrac{1}{2}\mathbf{G}_{ij} + 2\mathbf{CE}_{ij}, \\ \mathbf{DZW}_{ij} &= \mathbf{SE}_{ij} + \tfrac{1}{2}\mathbf{G}_{ij}, \end{aligned}$$

where SE_{ij} is the matrix of specific or within family environmental effects, CE_{ij} the matrix of common or family environmental effects, and G_{ij} the matrix of additive genetic effects.

This model is familiar enough and I do not wish to consider in detail the assumptions underlying it since they have been discussed elsewhere [Jinks and Fulker, 1970; Fulker, 1974]. Suffice it to say the model assumes only additive genetic variance, that genotype-environment covariance and interaction are both absent, and that MZ and DZ twins share relevant aspects of their environment to the same extent. These assumptions are frequently called into question; much less often are they demonstrated to be false. Only the last assumption is really critical and to my knowledge it has never been clearly demonstrated to be false in any study. Certainly MZ twins share more experiences than DZ twins, but whether these are experiences relevant to the trait in question is often doubtful. In my view, the model is a reasonable approximation for a number of physical and behavioral traits.

The problem of applying the multivariate analysis of variance approach to this model stems from the necessity to set up a proper F ratio which unambiguously establishes the effect in question. The ratio $(\mathbf{DZW})\,(\mathbf{MZW})^{-1}$ establishes the within-pair genetic variance, but no such ratio exists to cope with the common environmental component CE_{ij}. Neither can we, in the absence of CE_{ij}, combine all four observed mean cross product matrices to provide an overall estimate of the remaining components G_{ij} and E_{ij}.

One approach that promises to go some way towards overcoming these limitations is a maximum likelihood approach similar to that used by Taubman [1977] and that advocated by Martin and Eaves [1977]. This approach allows us to use all the available data efficiently and to explore the component structures systematically using χ^2 tests of significance to arrive at reasonable decisions.

We assume that the raw observations follow a bivariate normal distribution, so that the observed mean cross product matrices follow that of the Wishart. If these k matrices, the between and within matrices of twin analysis in the present case, are denoted S_{kij} or $\mathbf{S}_k$ for short, with expectations $E(\mathbf{S}_k)$, then the following expression provides a log-likelihood ratio statistic, F, following χ^2 in large samples. If we parameterize $E(\mathbf{S}_k)$ in terms of the required model and minimize the function with respect to these parameters, we obtain their maximum likelihood estimates. Only the χ^2 value is sensitive to the sample size, the estimates always being maximum likelihood.

$$F = \sum_{k=1}^{m} N_k \left\{ \ln |E(\mathbf{S}_k)| - \ln |\mathbf{S}_k| + \mathrm{tr}[\mathbf{S}_k E(\mathbf{S}_k)^{-1}] - P \right\},$$

where N_k = df of the k-th matrix and P = the number of variates. Functions such as these can now be minimized by a number of optimization routines available as packages through most university computing services. These routines frequently employ the first derivatives to minimize the function and the second derivatives to provide standard errors for the parameters, but numerical methods are usually optionally available to avoid the necessity for explicit differentiation. Supplying the derivatives often improves the efficiency of the routines, and Martin and Eaves [1977] offer these for the factor analysis model. The routines used in the present analyses were made available by CERN [1976], the European Centre for Nuclear Research.

Should we also wish to fit models that are not automatically constrained, the routines include procedures for specifiying rectangular constraints to keep parameters within upper and lower bounds, and more complex constraints may be forced by devising a penalty function in which the χ^2 value is augmented by a continuous positive function of the violated constraint. This function vanishes when the constraint is satisfied, leaving the required χ^2 goodness-of-fit statistic. In passing it is worth noting that the use of the above procedures make the constrained maximum likelihood estimation of components in univariate analyses so straightforward that there would appear to be no longer any justification for using more primitive unconstrained methods such as weighted least squares.

The main problems encountered in this approach are the problem of uniqueness general to multivariate analysis and the special problem of singularity that may result from forcing constraints once we stray from straightforward principal component models. The uniqueness problem has been thoroughly discussed by Jöreskog [1969] in the context of maximum likelihood factor analysis. Generally it may be overcome in orthogonal analyses by fixing certain component or factor loadings to zero so that the solution is unique. A simple transformation may be used to obtain the conventional loadings should these be desired, although the use of zero loadings may well help in exploring the covariance structure. In correlated factor analyses a second-order structure written onto the correlations between the factors can also be made to produce a unique solution. Exactly the same solutions may be adopted in the component analysis approach we are discussing.

The singularity problem caused by forcing simple constraints will usually be dealt with automatically by the minimization routine ensuring convergence, appropriate parameter estimates, and the χ^2 goodness-of-fit statistic. However, the matrix of second derivatives may become singular too, and standard errors unobtainable unless we subsequently fix certain parameter values. Taken together, these problems require that we feel our way in building up suitable models, and I would like to try to give something of the flavor of this approach with two simple examples.

The first example involves twin data collected by Zuckerman at the Institute of Psychiatry in London, using our volunteer twin register. His area of research is arousal and the need to seek stimulation, a characteristic he measures with a sensation-seeking questionnaire.

There are four subscales in the questionnaire, each measuring a different aspect of sensation seeking. One, Disinhibition (Dis) is concerned with seeking release through activities such as party going, social drinking, and sexual activities. Another, Thrill and Adventure Seeking (TAS) is concerned with a liking for dangerous and exciting sports. Experience Seeking (ES) involves novel sensations and unconventional experiences, mainly in the social context, while Boredom Susceptibility (BS) is concerned with intolerance of routine activities and dull, predictable people. Zuckerman [1974], reviewing a large body of research with the questionnaire, makes a case for individual differences in the average score on these scales, reflecting the need for different optimal levels of stimulation. He presents evidence implicating constitutional factors, such as levels of platelet monoamine oxidase (MAO), which correlate negatively with sensation seeking, gonadal hormones which correlate positively, the orienting reflex in response to novel stimuli, and the evoked cortical response in reaction to intense ones. As one might expect for such measures, there are marked sex and age differences. While young men frequently express a liking for skydiving and wild parties, most elderly ladies do not.

We [Fulker et al, 1976] decided to investigate the possibility of a constitutional basis for sensation seeking through a twin study of same-sex and opposite-sex twins. The questionnaire was mailed to 422 pairs of male and female twins, in the age range of 18 to 52 years. Scores were age-corrected by analysis of covariance and subscale variances standardized to unity across the whole sample. The comparability of subscale variances permitted univariate analysis of variance for taking a preliminary look at the the structure of the data, a useful procedure when one is trying to feel one's way with respect to an appropriate genetic and environmental model as well as an appropriate structural one.

Consequently we carried out a repeated measures analysis of variance both between and within pairs with individual differences in total scores providing the between subject mean squares, and differences in subscale profiles the mean squares within subjects. To each we fitted a simple univariate additive genetic model with no common environment, one which has been found to fit a number of personality variables [Jinks and Fulker, 1970; Eaves and Eysenck, 1975; Eaves, 1977]. As we can see from Table II the fit was very good for the total sensation-seeking score, and the narrow heritability of 58% was quite high for a personality variable. However, the repeated measures analysis to the right of the table indicates that this simple model was inadequate for the trait profiles, the residual χ^2 being highly significant. The main cause of the problem is not difficult to see, it being the low between pairs mean square for opposite sex DZ twins (DZ_{os}) which is virtually the same size as the mean square within, indicating zero resemblance for these pairs in spite of a moderate degree of resemblance for same-sex DZ pairs. This pattern suggests either different genes are controlling the profiles in men and women, or a form of sex x genotype interaction, the two being formally equivalent. A simplified form of sex interaction model is shown in Table II, apparently accounting for the data very well. Evidently there is a strong common genetic component in mean level of sensation seeking, but the genetic determination of the pattern that goes to make up a particular level is under different genetic control in the two sexes.

With a reasonable univariate genetic and environmental model we felt confident in fitting a multivariate extension to the ten 4 × 4 mean cross products

TABLE II. ANOVA of Sensation Seeking

| | | | | Total score analysis | | | | | Profile analysis | | | | |
| | | | | Model 1 | | | | | Model 1 | | Model 2 | | |
Twir	Item	df	MS	V(SE)	V(G)	df	MS	V(SE)	V(G)	V(SE)[a]	V(G)	V(G × S)
MZf	B	172	2.96	1	2	516	0.91	1	2	1	2	2
	W	174	0.83	1	0	522	0.37	1	0	1	0	0
MZm	B	57	3.57	1	2	171	1.17	1	2	1	2	2
	W	59	0.82	1	0	177	0.47	1	0	1	0	0
DZf	B	110	2.08	1	1½	330	0.80	1	1½	1	1½	1½
	W	112	1.35	1	½	336	0.47	1	½	1	½	½
DZm	B	24	2.30	1	1½	72	0.99	1	1½	1	1½	1½
	W	26	1.51	1	½	78	0.51	1	½	1	½	½
DZ$_{os}$	B	49	3.91	1	1½	147	0.64	1	1½	1	1½	1½
	W	50	1.55	1	½	150	0.76	1	½	1	½	1½
Estimates				0.83	1.16			0.41	0.29	0.41	0.18	0.43
χ^2				140.59*	23.36*			420.25*	33.64*	402.25*	2.68	15.28*
								$\chi^2_8 = 29.56*$		$\chi^2_7 = 8.52$		

Residual $\chi^2_8 = 8.59$

*P < 0.001.

[a] V(SE) in model 2 includes SE × sex interactions.

matrices calculated for the five twin groups. The form of the data, omitting the last eight matrices for convenience, together with the model, are shown in Table III.

Maximum likelihood estimates of the three component matrices are shown in Table IV. Initially, an unconstrained estimation procedure was used to see if constraints were necessary. The estimates of SE_{ij} and G_{ij} did, in fact, turn out to be Gramian, but the estimated SG_{ij} did not, one estimated correlation being -2.14. Consequently, a penalty function approach was used to obtain a constrained estimate of SG_{ij}, with the result shown at the foot of the table.

The form of the penalty function was

$$P = Q \sum_{i=1}^{n} \lambda_i^2.$$

The λ_i are the n negative latent roots of the estimated component matrix SG_{ij} at any given time during the minimization, and Q is an arbitrarily large constant modified as the minimization proceeds. The function minimized is the original maximum likelihood function plus P. By starting in a feasible region, where all the λ are positive, making Q progressively larger, and setting a very small limit to λ, most minimization routines, even using gradient methods, will find a satisfactory minimum.

In the present case the constrained estimate of SG_{ij} has three positive roots, the remaining one being nought. Such a matrix has only nine free elements, not ten as in the full rank case. With only nine free parameters one degree of freedom is therefore lost from the residual χ^2 giving a nonsignificant difference χ_1^2 of 1.47. Clearly the constraint not only produces a sensible estimate of SG_{ij} but is also fully consistent with the data. In either case, constrained or unconstrained, the residual χ^2 values indicate a very good fit of the interaction model.

The structure of these constrained component matrices could be explored successfully by any conventional multivariate technique. By inspection their form indicates a general factor for G_{ij}, all the correlations being positive, and a bipolar factor for SG_{ij} in view of both negative and positive correlations. This pattern is consistent with the univariate analysis in which the total score corresponds to the general factor controlled by additive genes, and the profile scores, which involve orthogonal contrasts with plus and minus signs, correspond to the bipolar factor controlled by different genes in the two sexes.

The exploratory approach to factor structures is difficult to combine with significance testing, especially in component analysis. Consequently, the direct structural approach involving a model consisting of factor loadings and specific variances fitted directly to the data was employed, but in a progressive manner to allow for tests of significance of successive aspects of the model. However,

TABLE III. Multivariate Model and ANCOVA: Sensation Seeking*

Twin	Item	Expectation	df	Mean cross products			
				Dis	TAS	ES	BS
MZf	B	$SE_{ij} + 2G_{ij} + 2SG_{ij}$	172	1.35	0.38	0.69	0.70
					1.49	0.64	0.24
						1.56	0.42
							1.29
MZf	W	SE_{ij}	174	0.47	0.12	0.17	0.16
					0.58	0.09	0.11
						0.42	0.04
							0.45
MZm	B	} as above	57				—
	W		59				—
DZf	B	$SE_{ij} + 1\frac{1}{2}G_{ij} + 1\frac{1}{2}SG_{ij}$	110				—
	W	$SE_{ij} + \frac{1}{2}G_{ij} + \frac{1}{2}SG_{ij}$	112				—
DZm	B	} as above	24				—
	W		26				—
DZ$_{OS}$	B	$SE_{ij} + 1\frac{1}{2}G_{ij} + \frac{1}{2}SG_{ij}$	49				—
	W	$SE_{ij} + \frac{1}{2}G_{ij} + 1\frac{1}{2}SG_{ij}$	50				—

*SE_{ij}, specific environmental covariance matrix; G_{ij}, additive genetic covariance matrix; SG_{ij}, additive genetic × sex interaction covariance matrix. Sensation-seeking scales: Dis, Disinhibition; TAS, Thrill and Adventure Seeking; ES, Experience Seeking; BS, Boredom Susceptibility.

TABLE IV. Solution to ANCOVA Sensation Seeking

	Components				Correlations				Residual χ^2
	Dis	TAS	ES	BS					
SE_{ij}	0.46	0.13	0.16	0.16	1.00	0.26	0.36	0.33	
		0.56	0.10	0.07		1.00	0.20	0.13	
			0.44	0.05			1.00	0.11	
				0.50				1.00	
G_{ij}	0.88	0.18	0.41	0.57	1.00	0.26	0.42	0.71	
		0.55	0.46	0.05		1.00	0.60	0.08	
			1.08	0.67			1.00	0.75	
				0.73				1.00	
SG_{ij}	0.17	-0.03	0.10	0.05	1.00	-0.12	0.82	0.23	$\chi^2_{70} = 73.62$ ns
		0.36	0.06	0.11		1.00	0.50	0.34	
			0.04	-0.23			1.00	-2.14	
				0.29				1.00	
SG_{ij} constrained	0.15	-0.05	0.06	0.03	1.00	-0.22	0.44	0.13	$\chi^2_{71} = 75.09$ ns
		0.35	0.03	0.09		1.00	0.22	0.39	
			0.15	-0.16			1.00	-0.70	
				0.34				1.00	

no structure beyond the ten SE_{ij} was fitted to the environmental component since these influences are confounded with sex χ environmental interaction in these data.

The results are shown in Table V together with an approximate analysis of χ^2. The addition of each of the two factors and the specific variances produces a large reduction in χ^2, establishing the statistical significance of all these structural components. The full model in line 4 of the table provides a nonsignificant residual $\chi^2_{78} = 85.45$ indicating a satisfactory fit. The differences between this model and the full unconstrained covariance model shown in the final line of the table is not significant ($\chi^2_8 = 11.73$), indicating that the reduced rank model, involving 12 genetic parameters, explains the data as well as the full rank model involving 20. The pattern of loadings for the additive genetic component z_1, given at the foot of the table, confirms the presence of a strong general factor common to men and women, and the bipolar pattern of loadings for the interactive component p_i confirms the sex difference in the genetic determination of trait profiles. Genes that make for high TAS and ES and low Dis and BS in men appear to produce opposite effects in women.

TABLE V. Multivariate Model of Sensation Seeking†

Model	Resid χ^2	df	Diff χ^2	df
SE_{ij}	346.48*	90		
SE_{ij} ; $G_{ij} = z_i z_j$	242.26*	86	104.22*	4
SE_{ij} ; $G_{ij} = z_i z_j$; $S \times G_{ij} = p_i p_j$	163.01*	82	79.25*	4
SE_{ij} ; $G_{ij} = z_i z_j + (s_i^2$ when $i = j$); $S \times G_{ij} = p_i p_j$	85.45	78	77.56*	4
SE_{ij} ; G_{ij} ; $S \times G_{ij}$	73.62	70	11.73	8

	Estimate of Genetic Parameters		
	Additive		Additive $\times$ sex
	z_i	s_i	p_i
Dis	0.63	0.75	0.27
TAS	0.45	0.78	-0.27
ES	0.93	0.36	-0.35
BS	0.71	0.38	0.59
Genetic variance	49%	36%	15%

*$p < 0.001$.

†z_i, Loadings of general additive genetic factor; s_i, specific variances of additive genetic factor; p_i, loadings on additive $\times$ sex interaction factor. Resid, Residual; Diff, Difference, here and in Table VI.

Since the former traits involve socially acceptable forms of activity, and the latter include activities which are less socially acceptable, it is perhaps not surprising, even today, that genes controlling these measures should express themselves differently in men and women.

One further analysis was carried out to see if the structure of the environmental component was similar to the genetic component, even given the confounding of sex interaction effects with those of the specific environment. The DZ_{os} twins were dropped from the analysis and a simple SE_{ij}, G_{ij} model fitted to the twins of the same sex, these parameters being understood to represent a main effect confounded with sex interaction, in accordance with the expectations in Table III. In order to test the equality of the two covariance structures, G_{ij} was reparameterized as a weighted composite of SE_{ij},

$$G_{ij} = w_i w_j SE_{ij}.$$

If this model should fit, identical correlation structures for G_{ij} and SE_{ij} are implied.

The results are shown in Table VI. Clearly the hypothesis of equality of correlational structures is supported, especially if we allow for specific variation,

TABLE VI. Testing Genetic and Environmental Correlations Having Same Structures: Sensation Seeking†

Model for like-sexed twins	Resid χ^2	df	Diff χ^2	df
SE_{ij} ; $G_{ij} = w_i w_j SE_{ij}$	82.82	66		
SE_{ij} ; $G_{ij} = w_i w_j \left\{ SE_{ij} - (s_i^2 \text{ when } i = j) \right\}$	64.63	62	18.19*	4
SE_{ij} ; G_{ij}	61.61	60	3.02	2

	First two orthogonal components				Error variance	
	1st	2nd	Resid	s_i^2	reported	$h^2 = w_i^2/(1 + w_i^2)$
Dis	0.84	0.37		0.00	0.19	53%
TAS	0.56	−0.63		0.19	0.34	55%
ES	0.85	−0.33		0.30	0.23	80%
BS	0.74	0.43		0.36	0.38	79%
Genetic variance	58%	22%	20%			

*p < 0.002.

†$w_i w_j$, the relative weight of G_{ij} to SE_{ij} element for element; s_i^2, variance specific to SE_{ij} when $i = j$.

s_i^2, in the environmental component. The values of s_i^2 are similar to the error variation quoted for these tests and probably represent the same source of variation. Analysis of this common genetic and environmental component reveals a very similar general and bipolar structure to that previously found. This finding may indicate that genetic and environmental influences for these measures have similar underlying mechanisms.

Next I would like to consider a rather different example involving a re-analysis of Taubman's [1977] twin study of schooling, income, and occupational status. This study probably represents the most extensive and sophisticated example of structural genetic component analysis available to date, as well as being of great substantive interest.

One question raised by his analysis with Behrman and Wales [Behrman et al, 1977] was why a model involving only one environmental component was used throughout. Inspection of their table of cross-sib correlations for MZ and DZ twins indicated a common environmental covariance matrix (estimated as twice the DZ correlations minus the MZ correlations, in the conventional manner) with one negative variance, three undefined correlations, and three correlations greater than 1. This component was clearly far from Gramian in form, strongly suggesting the necessity for a reduced rank model of common environment.

However, these effects might simply have been the result of sampling variation, so the MZ and DZ correlations were converted to mean cross products and subjected to the constrained maximum likelihood estimation procedure. Since Taubman's original analysis had the form of a kind of path analysis, it was decided to reparameterize the component covariance matrices as variances and correlations to facilitate further investigation. For example, G_{ij}, was replaced by $RG_{ij}G_i^{1/2}G_j^{1/2}$, where the RG_{ij} are the correlations and the G_i factors the variances. The Gramian constraint was ensured in two ways. Firstly, rectangular constraints were applied to all the parameters so that the variances could not become negative and the correlations were bounded by ± 1. Secondly, the latent roots of the covariance matrices were all required to be $\geqslant 0$ by means of a penalty function.

The estimated component correlation matrices, together with the components of variances as percentages, are shown in Table VII. The model fits quite well, especially when we consider the power of the test with sample sizes around 4,000. The choice of a single variable for common environment appears to be forced by the data exactly as it was in Tukey's analysis, the unitary values in the correlation matrix indicating the necessity of a single rank model. There appears to be only one common environmental influence general to schooling and subsequent adult status and income, an influence which it seems plausible to equate with the environmental effects of social origins.

One problem with the simple twin model, as soon as we wish to include common environment, is that we can no longer be sure that the effects of nonadditive gene action, assortative mating, and the correlated genetic and environmental influences

TABLE VII. Constrained Parameter Estimates: Taubman's Twin Study [1977]†

		Correlations			Variances (%)
		Specific Environment (SE)			
Schooling (S)	1.00	0.17	0.24	0.10	23
Occupation 1 (O_1)		1.00	0.17	0.07*	48
Occupation 2 (O_2)			1.00	0.14	64
Income (I)				1.00	45
		Genetic (G)			
	1.00	0.60	0.62	0.55	46
		1.00	0.63	0.52	33
			1.00	0.44	28
				1.00	47
		Common Environment (CE)			
	1.00	1.00	1.00	1.00	31
		1.00	1.00	1.00	19*
			1.00	1.00	8*
				1.00	8*

*p < 0.01; for all others p < 0.001.
†Residual $\chi^2_{16} = 24.99$, p < 0.1.

are absent. If present, they bias the estimate of common environment, decreasing it in the case of nonadditivity and being completely confounded with it in the other two cases [Jinks and Fulker, 1970; Fulker, 1974].

Taubman attempts to explore these problems by freeing the DZ genetic correlations ρ from the value of 0.5, which the simple twin model assumes, allowing it to take its own value in the estimation procedure. He found a value of about 0.35 to be consistent with the data, implying considerable nonadditive genetic variation, although a distinct possibility in this particular study was a restricted sampling of family influences. However, with his approach the estimate of common environment is still confounded with assortative mating which, in turn, will force the genetic correlation to become unrealistically low. In addition a single value of ρ might not be realistic if the degree of assortative mating and nonadditive gene action should differ between measures, as might well be true.

To explore these possibilities, the following model was adopted which allowed for a separate sib genetic correlation for each measure (ρ_i):

$$MZB_{ij} = SE_{ij} + 2G_{ij} + 2CE_{ij},$$

$$MZW_{ij} = SE_{ij},$$

$$DZB_{ij} = SE_{ij} + (1 + \rho_i^{\frac{1}{2}} \rho_j^{\frac{1}{2}})G_{ij} + 2CE_{ij},$$

$$DZW_{ij} = SE_{ij} + (1 - \rho_i^{\frac{1}{2}} \rho_j^{\frac{1}{2}})G_{ij}.$$

Parameters estimated by the constrained procedure are given in Table VIII for three different models. Model 1 is the simple model previously fitted with all values of ρ_i fixed at 0.5 and a single common environment. That is, the conventional twin model fits quite well. Model 2 frees the four ρ values but retains a single common environment. This model gives a slightly better fit (the difference χ_4^2 being 9.64, $P \simeq 0.05$), and some of the values of ρ_i are improbably low. The similarity of the estimates in all other respects, together with the merely modest improvement in fit, clearly indicates the data are relatively insensitive to the values of the sib genetic correlation. Put differently, the joint test that the ρ values differ from 0.5 barely reaches the 0.05 probability level.

In both these models the effects of assortative mating are still confounded with common environment, even though ρ has taken account of nonadditive gene action. However, if we drop common environment from the model but still keep the ρ values free, to give model 3, the effect of assortative mating is accommodated by the ρ values in addition to the effect of nonadditive gene action. These additional effects may be seen in the increased estimates of ρ. Now, though, the model fails quite badly, the residual χ_{16}^2 being 40.63, $P < 0.001$. Clearly a model assuming no common environment is quite unrealistic, even allowing for assortative mating, nonadditivity and possible restricted sampling. Since if there is at least some common environment, its component must be at least rank one, and something between model 1 and 2 would seem to be required by the data. As the χ^2 values and the estimates of the variances differ only slightly between these two models, parsimony favors the conventional model 1. Probably, as appears to be true for IQ [Jinks and Fulker, 1970], assortative mating and nonadditivity balance out, making a ρ of 0.5 quite a realistic assumption.

Bearing in mind the limitation that common environmental effects may still include some effects of correlated genes and environment, we can explore the structure of the component variances and correlations in model 1 further (shown in Table VII) by means of the modified path model shown in Figure 1.

In this model only three of the four variables have been selected for analysis since they can be plausibly related longitudinally. These are schooling (S) and the two measures relating to the individual some 30 years later, namely, occupational status (Oc_2) and income (Inc). On the left of the figure are the three influences G, SE, and CE that affect schooling. These influences are also assumed to affect income and status some 30 years later. However, in addition income and status are assumed to be influenced by the residual genetic and environmental effects shown in the right of the figure. No residual common environment is needed in view of the rank one structure of this component. Following the conventions of path analysis [Wright, 1954], the casual influences of the seven latent variables on the three measures S, Inc, and Oc_2 are represented by straight arrows bearing the path coefficients that indicate their relative influence when all the other

TABLE VIII. Taubman's [1977] Data: Different Sib Genetic Correlations

		% Variances			ρ_i	χ^2	df	P
		SE	G	CE				
Model 1 all $\rho_i = 0.5$, $RCE_{ij} = 1.0$	S	23	46	31	0.50	24.99	16	< 0.1
	O_1	48	33	19	0.50			
	O_2	64	28	8	0.50			
	I	45	47	8	0.50			
Model 2 all ρ_i free, $RCE_{ij} = 1.0$	S	18	45	37	0.19	15.35	12	ns
	O_1	36	46	18	0.33			
	O_2	50	40	11	0.15			
	I	31	61	8	0.42			
Model 3 all ρ_i free, no CE	S	13	87	0	0.67	40.63	16	< 0.001
	O_1	30	70	0	0.68			
	O_2	47	53	0	0.56			
	I	29	71	0	0.55			

[a]ρ_i, Genetic sib correlation for i-th measure.

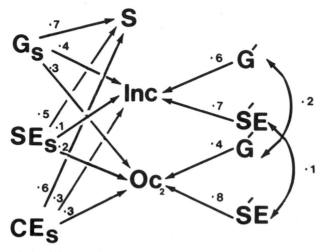

Fig 1. Path analysis of Taubman's [1977] twin study. Latent variables: G_S, genetic influences on schooling; SE_S, specific environmental influences on schooling; CE_S, common family influences on schooling; G^1, residual genetic influences; SE^1, residual specific environmental influences. Observed variables: S, schooling (years); Inc, adult income (log $); Oc_2, adult occupational status.

factors in the system are held constant. The relationships between the residual effects are represented by curved arrows simply indicating the existence of a correlation. Coefficients have been rounded to one decimal place for simplicity.

This diagram indicates aspects of the genetic and environmental influences on adult status and income, not all of which are obvious from simple inspection of the correlations and variances given in Table VII. Most of these conclusions follow from Taubman's analysis too, but the path diagram has the advantage of providing a convenient summary.

Firstly, both genes and common environment for schooling subsequently influence adult status and income, roughly to the same extent, all four paths being between 0.3 and 0.4. Secondly, specific environmental effects on schooling, that is, chance and accidental factors, exert an almost trivial influence later, their paths being between 0.1 and 0.2. Thirdly, by far the greatest influences on adult income and status are residual genetic and specific environmental factors. Fourthly, these strong residual factors are largely independent of each other with respect to the two adult measures, their correlations being merely 0.1 and 0.2.

This analysis suggests, then, that insofar as schooling influences adult status, home environment is almost as important as genetic endowment, but that large independent genetic and environmental influences unrelated to home environment play the major role. One could hazard a guess that these later genetic influences are related more to temperament and special skills than to IQ, which we know has a powerful influence on schooling. The environmental factors probably relate to market imperfections and luck.

These two examples have, I hope, indicated something of the scope of the maximum likelihood approach to the multivariate structural analysis of genetic and environmental influences using twins. It could, of course, be extended with no difficulty to include additional kinships. It is possible to handle a variety of models and the method is probably statistically optimal. Its only drawback seems to be the demands it makes on computer time, and the development of more efficient algorithms geared to the needs of particular problems can be expected to remove this limitation.

ACKNOWLEDGMENTS

I would like to thank Owen White for generously sharing with me his extensive knowledge of multivariate analysis and optimization. I would also like to thank Nick Martin and Lindon Eaves for many helpful discussions.

REFERENCES

Bartlett MS (1951): The goodness of fit of a single hypothetical discriminant function in the case of several groups. Ann Eugen 16:199–214.

Behrman J, Taubman P, Wales T (1977): Controlling for and measuring the effects of genetic and family environment in equations for schooling and labour market success. In Taubman P (ed): "Kinometrics: The Determinants of Socioeconomic Success Within and Between Families." Amsterdam: North Holland.

Bock RD, Petersen AC (1975): A multivariate correction for attenuation. Biometrika 62(3): 673–678.

Bock RD, Vandenberg SG (1968): Components of heritable variation in mental test scores. In Vandenberg SG (ed): "Progress in Human Behavior Genetics." Baltimore: Johns Hopkins University Press.

CERN (1974): Minuit; A package of programs to minimise a function of a variable, compute the covariance matrix and find the true errors. Geneva, Switzerland: CERN.

Eaves LJ (1973): The structure of genotypic and environmental covariation for personality measurements: An analysis of the PEN. Br J Soc Clin Psychol 12:275–828.

Eaves LJ (1977): Inferring the causes of human variation. J Roy Statist Soc A 140:123–146.

Eaves LJ, Eysenck HJ (1975): The nature of extraversion: A genetical analysis. J Pers Soc Psychol 32:102–112.

Fulker DW (1974): Applications of biometrical genetics to human behaviour. In van Abeelen JHF (ed): "The Genetics of Behaviour." Amsterdam: North Holland.

Fulker DW, Zuckerman M, Eysenck SB (1976): A genetic and environmental analysis of sensation seeking. Mimeo. Dept of Psychology, Institute of Psychiatry, London.

Jinks JL, Fulker DW (1970): Comparison of the biometrical genetical, MAVA, and classical approaches to the analysis of human behaviour. Psychol Bull 73:311–349.

Jöreskog KG (1969): A general approach to confirmatory maximum likelihood factor analysis. Psychometrika 34:183–202.

Kempthorne O, Osborne RH (1961): The interpretation of twin data. Am J Hum Genet 13:320–329.

Loehlin JC, Vandenberg SG (1968): Genetic and environmental components in the covariation of cognitive abilities: An additive model. In Vandenberg SG (ed): "Progress in Human Behavior Genetics." Baltimore: Johns Hopkins University Press.

Martin NG, Eaves LJ (1977): The genetical analysis of covariance structure. Heredity 38: 79–95.

Nance WE, Nakata M, Paul TD, Yu P (1974): The use of twin studies in the analysis of phenotypic traits in man. In Janevich DT, Skalko RG, Porter IH (eds): "Congenital Defects. New Directions in Research." New York: Academic Press.

Taubman P (ed) (1977): "Kinometrics: The Determinants of Socioeconomic Success Within and Between Families." Amsterdam: North Holland.

Tukey JW (1951): Components in regression. Biometrics 7:33–69.

Wright S (1954): The interpretation of multivariate systems. In Kempthorne O, Bancroft TA, Gowen JW, Lush JL (eds): "Statistics and Mathematics in Biology." Ames, Iowa: Iowa State College Press.

Zuckerman M (1974): The sensation seeking motive. In Maher B (ed): "Progress in Experimental Personality Research." London: Academic Press.

Multivariate Analysis in Twin Studies

E Defrise-Gussenhoven and C Susanne

In multivariate analysis, many characters are used simultaneously and twin differences can be studied in terms of measured distances. For biometric characters, generalized distances have yielded results which have seemed in accordance with the polygenic model [Defrise-Gussenhoven, 1967; Vrydagh-Laoureux and Defrise-Gussenhoven, 1971; Susanne, 1974]. We shall first give a summary of these results. Then we will introduce distances for qualitative characters, and use them in the question of uniovular dispermatic twins.

1. TYPES OF TWINS AND NOTATION

Identical twins (IT) are identical for sex and for the qualitative characters depending on major genes used in the study. If many characters have been used, the chance that they are monozygotic is practically 100%.

Nonidentical twins (NIT) consist of DZT and three hypothetical cases — POT, SOT, and UDT [Mysberg, 1957; Weninger, 1961].

Dizygotic twins (DZT) result from the fertilization by two spermatozoa of two maternal cells arisen from different primary oocytes. Their genetic difference is the same as that of ordinary sibs (see end of section 4).

Primary oocytary twins (POT) result when two maternal cells arise from one primary oocyte. These twins are as dissimilar as DZT.

Secondary oocytary twins (SOT) result from a secondary oocyte, when an ovum and a giant secondary polar body arise; both cells are fertilized by separate spermatozoa. When the mother is heterozygotic for a given locus and when there is prereduction, the twins will receive the same genes from the mother; but when there is crossing-over and postreduction, the twins will receive different genes from the mother. In the first case, the partners will be more similar, in the second

Twin Research: Psychology and Methodology, pages 237–243

case less similar than DZT; everything depends on the position of the locus and the number of crossing-overs. In this paper, we assume that since many loci are considered, the results of the two situations cancel each other out and that on the whole SOT are just as dissimilar as DZT.

Uniovular dispermatic twins (UDT) result when an ordinary haploid ovum undergoes an extra mitotic division, each of the daughter cells being fertilized by a separate spermatozoa. UDT receive the same genes from a heterozygotic mother; they are more similar than DZT.

$$\alpha = P(UDT/NIT) = \text{the probability that NIT are UDT.}$$

2. GENERALIZED DISTANCES FOR BIOMETRIC CHARACTERS IN SAME-SEX TWIN PAIRS

For several groups of biometric characters generalized distances between IT and NIT were compared [Vrydagh-Laoureux and Defrise-Gussenhoven, 1971]. If C denotes the covariance matrix of a normal p-variate population, and a,b the vectors having as elements the measurement of two subjects, A,B, belonging to this population, then

$$\Delta(A,B) = [(a - b)' \, C^{-1} \, (a - b)]^{1/2}$$

is the generalized distance between A and B. If A and B are not related and if there are n such randomly chosen pairs A,B, then

$$x = [\Sigma\Delta^2 (A,B)]^{1/2}$$

is normally distributed with $m = (2np - 1)^{1/2}$ as mean and 1 as variance.

For $p = 4$ measurements, the 30 IT had $x = 6.17$, whereas the expected mean for random pairs was $m = 15.46$. The difference (9.29), more than 9 times the standard deviation, indicates that IT are extremely similar for head measurements.

In Figure 1, results for head, body, and face are compared with the following results: a) IT and NIT resemble each other more than random pairs; b) IT are more similar than NIT; c) the similarity of IT tends to increase as more measurements are used; d) the difference between the groups of IT and NIT is greatest for the body; e) NIT are strikingly similar for the face (see Defrise-Gussenhoven [1970]); this resemblance makes the hypothesis of the existence of UDT reasonable.

Susanne [1974] using the same method in families, found manifest assortative mating and greater sib-sib than NIT distances for head and face, although the contrary was true for the body.

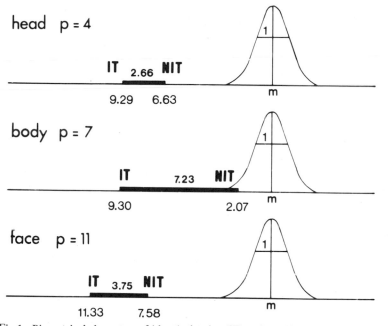

Fig 1. Biometrical characters of identical twins (IT) and nonidentical twins (NIT).

3. ESTIMATION OF α = P(UDT/NIT)

When qualitative characters such as blood groups, immunoglobulins, hapto-globins, and HLA system depend on major genes, each can be used to estimate α in a group of NIT. For instance, supposing random mating and denoting by p and q the frequencies of the genes M and N, the probability of equal genotypes in NIT is easily seen to be

$$P = (p^4 + 2p^3q + 3.5p^2q^2 + 2pq^3 + q^4)$$
$$+ \alpha(p^3q + 0.5p^2q^2 + pq^3).$$

In a sample of 244 pairs, Schiff and von Verschuer [1933] found 62.3% with identical genotypes for the MN blood group. Taking $\hat{p} = 0.546$, the frequency of M in the 244 pairs, and equating P to 0.623, we find $\hat{\alpha} = 0.171$, a rough estimate of α.

For each character, an estimation of α can be made by this method. We have calculated the theoretical P values for genotypes or phenotypes with three alleles for a locus. Generalization to more than four alleles is immediate (but the formulas are long!). However, since for each estimate the information of only one character is used, we prefer a more powerful method to test the existence of UDT; this is given in section 4.

4. DISTANCES DEPENDING ON GENOTYPES OR PHENOTYPES

There is a fairly large variety of such distances (Jacquard [1974] ; Corluy [1977]), the choice depending on the aim one has in view. The weighted distances for several loci can be added, the sum D again being a distance storing a great deal of information.

For blood group MN, we denote by d_{12}, d_{13}, d_{23} the distances between the genotypes MM-MN, MM-NN, and MN-NN. The choice of the distance functions is discussed in section 5.

Let A_i, B_i, C_i denote three members of the i-th of n families, A_i and B_i being NIT and C_i one of their sibs. For each pair of sibs, the distance, depending on the genotypes, is noted.

The expected mean values of the distances are easily seen to be

$$E\{d(A,C)\} = E\{d(B,C)\} = d_{12}(2p^3q + p^2q^2) + d_{13}(0.5p^2q^2)$$

$$+ d_{23}(2pq^3 + p^2q^2),$$

because A,C and B,C are ordinary sibs.

$$E\{d(A,B)\} = E\{d(A,C)\} - \alpha\{d_{12}p^3q + d_{13}(0.5p^2q^2) + d_{23}pq^3\},$$

which shows that, as soon as $\alpha \neq 0$, the expected distance for NIT will be smaller than for sibs.

If many genotypes or phenotypes are known, D is calculated for the three pairs of sibs of each family.

$$x_{i1} = D(A_i,B_i), \; x_{i2} = D(A_i,C_i), \; x_{i3} = D(B_i,C_i)$$

for $i = 1, 2, \ldots, n$, A being the elder twin.

An analysis of variance is performed with two controlled factors: 1) the families and 2) the type of relationship among the members of a family. It is this second factor which will be tested. The first factor is controlled in order to eliminate from the general variance eventual family effects such as serologic incompatibility of the parents or assortative mating. The model is, with $j = 1,2,3$,

$$x_{ij} = \mu + \mu_i + \nu_j + z_{ij};$$

μ is the general mean; μ_i the effect of the i-th family; ν_j the effect on x_{ij} of the j-th relationship; $\nu_2 = \nu_3$ because the distances between C and each of the twins have equal expectations; since $\nu_1 + \nu_2 + \nu_3 = 0$, we have also $\nu_1 = -2\nu_2$; z_{ij} is a normal random variable, with zero mean and variance σ^2. Randomness and normality are assumed because x_{ij} are linear functions of many random variables, the individual distances for each blood group.

The sums of squares

$$Q_2 = n \sum_{j=1}^{3} (x_{\cdot j} - x_{\cdot\cdot})^2 \text{ and } Q_1 = \sum_{j=1}^{3} \sum_{i=1}^{n} (x_{ij} - x_{\cdot j} - x_{i\cdot} + x_{\cdot\cdot})^2,$$

divided by their degrees of freedom 2 and $2(n-1)$, have expected values equal to $\sigma^2 + 3n\nu_2^2$ and σ^2. When

$$F_c = \frac{Q_2/2}{Q_1/2(n-1)} > F_{0.01},$$

the null hypothesis $\nu_2 = 0$ is rejected and the existence of UDT can be accepted.

Stern [1960] mentions NIT possessing more often the same ABO group than expected by chance; he suggests that this could be brought about by selective survival if both twins were compatible with the mother or even if they were compatible with each other. However, since many characters ought to be used in the analysis of variance presented in this section, we do not think that incompatibility for a few characters can greatly influence the results. Moreover, by controlling the first factor, we partly eliminate the effects of incompatibility of mother and children.

5. CHOICE OF DISTANCES

Many different distance functions between genotypes or phenotypes can be chosen and their efficiency compared. In Corluy [1977], qualities of several distances are discussed. One of these qualities states that a distance between two subjects must be smaller when they possess a common gene than when this is not the case. This propriety will tend to decrease the D value for UDT, because they share more often a common gene (received from a heterozygous mother) than other NIT. The Minkowski distance possesses this propriety; it is very flexible, because it can be used when not all the antisera are available or when no clear-cut genetic model yet exists, as is the case for the HLA system and a few others. Another advantage of the Minkowski distance is that it is not a function of the gene frequencies and that random mating must not be supposed.

The subjects are given scores 1 or 0 for positive or negative reactions. Then, for each character, the absolute differences of scores of two subjects are added and multiplied by the corresponding weight (Table I). D is the sum of these products. For instance, for A_i and B_i,

$$D(A_i,B_i) = \{|1-1| + |0-1|\}w_1 + \{|1-1| + |1-0| + |0-0|\}w_2 +$$

$$.. + \{|1-1| + |1-1| + |1-0| + |1-1| + |1-1|\}w_m$$

$$= w_1 + w_2 + \ldots + w_m.$$

These values are used in the analysis of variance of section 4.

The weights can be chosen equal to one, but also as a function of the information yielded by the reactions of the subjects to the antisera. For instance, with the antisera anti-A and anti-B we can have four combinations, whereas with anti-M and anti-N only three combinations are possible. Therefore, the blood group ABO can be given a greater weight than the blood group MN. A good choice of weights will increase the sensibility of the distance D.

Whenever biometric data exist, the sum $d = \Delta + D$ can be used in the analysis of variance and the results compared with those found with D alone.

TABLE I. Minkowski Distance With m Blood Groups: Scores for the Twins A_i,B_i and Their Sib C_i

Weight	w_1			w_2			w_m			
Blood group	MN			ABO			Rhesus			
antiserum	M	N	A	A_1	B	D	C	E	c	e
scores of A_i	1	0	1	1	0	1	1	1	1	1
scores of B_i	1	1	1	0	0	1	1	0	1	1
scores of C_i	0	1	1	0	1	1	1	1	0	0

$$D(A_i,B_i) = \{|1-1| + |0-1|\}w_1 + \{|1-1| + |1-0| + |0-0|\}w_2 +$$

$$.. + \{|1-1| + |1-1| + |1-0| + |1-1| + |1-1|\}w_m$$

REFERENCES

Corluy R (1977): Genetische afstanden tussen individuen gebaseerd op kwalitatieve gegevens. Doctoral dissertation. Brussels: Vrije Universiteit Brussel.

Defrise-Gussenhoven E (1967): Generalized distance in twin studies. Acta Genet (Basel) 17:275–288.

Defrise-Gussenhoven E (1970): Multivariate analysis in twins. Acta Genet Med Gemellol (Roma) 19:150–154.

Methodological Issues in Twin Research: The Assumption of Environmental Equivalence

Eleanor Dibble, Donald J Cohen, and Jane M Grawe

The twin intrapair comparative method provides a unique and valuable way for studying traits and diseases in man because of the opportunity it offers for exploring interactions between genetic endowment and environmental influences. The use of twin methodology is based on the assumptions that the zygosity of the twins has been correctly determined and that the environmental influence is the same for each co-twin, for each type of twinship and, for generalization, for twins and singletons. Our research with a large sample of twins (N — 377) in vestigating childhood personality determinants offers additional understanding of these issues by providing a new, tested method of zygosity determination and data which can be examined for common prenatal and postnatal environment variances.

Assignment of zygosity is fundamental to twin research. Those familiar with the literature are aware that although Galton [1875] assumed there were two distinct types of twins in his nature-nuture studies, the criteria for distinguishing one type from the other have not been consistent over time nor highly reliable. Twin research published prior to 1925 generally held that monozygotic twins were invariably enclosed in a single chorion, dizygotic in double chorions. The number of chorions was the absolute criterion for determining zygosity [Osborne, 1955]. However, not only was data on fetal membranes usually unavailable in obstetrical records, but Corner [1955], among others, proved this method to be invalid in many instances. Siemens' [1927] four levels of similarity method became the principal approach to zygosity assignment after 1925, although it was criticized for subjective bias in rating characteristics.

Today, tissue typing and blood factor analysis offer the greatest security for diagnosing zygosity; however, in epidemiological and other types of psychological research, especially involving children, there are often insurmountable constraints in obtaining blood specimens or performing the more elegant tissue transplanting procedures. Investigators have thus been forced to rely on other methods for

Twin Research: Psychology and Methodology, pages 245—251

zygosity assignment, including self-reports, clinical impressions, questionnaires, palmprints and statistical estimates [Bulmer, 1970; Cederlöf et al, 1961; Husen, 1959; Nichols and Bilbro, 1966].

In our epidemiological research on children's personality development, we have devised a new questionnaire type instrument which validly and reliably discriminates monozygotic (MZ) from dizygotic (DZ) twinships with an error rate which appears to approach that of blood typing. The questionnaire, completed by parents, consists of ten questions derived from clinical observations and previous studies. Six of the questions concern the degree to which the children are similar for specific physical characteristics, rated on a 3-point scale: "Not at all similar," 1; and "exactly similar or identical," 2. Four questions involve general identity and confusion scored dichotomously: "No" 0; or "yes" 1. All ten variables are assumed to be continuous but discrete measurement scales are used for ease of administration. (Table I lists the characteristics and social confusion question as well as the results of the reliability testing.)

The questionnaire instrument was tested for reliability with two groups of same-sex twins known to the Louisville Twin Research Project [Wilson, 1970] for whom blood typing for zygosity had been performed. At the time of their completion of the instruments, mothers from group A knew the zygosity assignment from blood typing and mothers from group B did not.

The zygosity questionnaire was analyzed in relation to the effect of mothers' prior knowledge of zygosity (from blood typing) and the effect of the children's age using the Hotelling's T^2 statistic as well as item-by-item analysis of variance. On the basis of these analyses it was evident that neither prior knowledge nor child age significantly altered parental response. There was no significant difference in parental responses for either MZ or DZ twinships in groups A and B.

In the assignment of a twinship to a zygosity group, there is little problem for twins who are rated "not at all similar" or "no" on all questions, or for twinships consistently rated at the opposite pole. However, for those twinships not close to the MZ and DZ extreme values, the complex relations between contributing variables must be weighted and assessed. Discriminant analysis, which produces weightings of variables contributing to a separation between groups, is well-suited to this purpose. Using discriminant analysis, MZ and DZ twins were clearly separated on the basis of all ten variables taken together and each variable was weighted. Assignment was in error in fewer than 3% of cases, closely approximating the results of routine blood typing procedures for zygosity assignment [Cohen et al, 1973, 1975].

From a substantive point of view, these studies highlight the differences in the environmental experiences of MZ and DZ twinships. For example, on questions concerning confusion, mothers rated 78% of MZ and 10% of DZ as experiencing confusion by mother and father, and 99% of MZ and 16% of DZ as experiencing confusion by strangers. The impact of such repeated confusion on individual

TABLE I. Zygosity Questionnaire Replies by Blood Type, %*

To what extent are the twins similar at this time for the following features?	Dizygotic twins N = 61				Monozygotic twins N = 94			
	Not at all similar	Somewhat similar	Exactly similar	Not at all similar	Somewhat similar	Exactly similar
Height	36.1	59.0	4.9	3.2	53.2	43.6
Weight	44.3	52.5	3.3	4.3	56.4	39.4
Facial appearance	68.9	31.1	0	0	44.7	55.3
Hair color	41.0	49.2	9.8	0	0	100
Eye color	34.4	47.5	18.0	0	1.1	98.9
Complexion	41.0	52.5	6.6	0	2.1	07.9
For each of the following check yes or no						
		No	Yes		No	Yes
Do they look as alike as two peas in a pod?		100	0		53.2	46.8
Does either mother or father ever confuse them?		90.2	9.8		22.3	77.7
Are they sometimes confused by other people in family?		85.3	14.8		6.4	93.6
Is it hard for strangers to tell them apart?		83.6	16.4		1.1	98.9

*Percentage are rounded off to nearest 0.1%.

twinships, or the effect of these differences between MZ and DZ twins is not known with certainty. However, such information must cast doubt upon the assumption of environmental equivalence.

Issues concerning environmental equivalence arise, also, well before the babies are born and during the first weeks of life. In our epidemiological studies, we have developed various questionnaire-type intruments for parental completion concerning parental perceptions of children's behavior [Cohen et al, 1977a], parents' interactions with their children [Cohen et al, 1977b], family stress [Dibble et al, 1976], and events and factors concerning children's gestation, delivery, and early psychological competence. In this report, we will focus on information in this last domain (Pregnancy, Delivery, and First Month of Life; PDF). Our major emphasis will be on the explication of environmental influences — both in utero and perinatal — which may have later impact on development and which may be relevant to the definition of environmental equivalence for MZ and DZ twinships and for twinships and singletons. The importance of such considerations for theoretical discussions of behavior genetics is apparent. For example, it has been repeatedly noted [eg, Husen, 1959] that twin populations appear to be more vulnerable to mental deficiency than singletons and that this phenomenon must be taken into consideration in generalizing twin data to singletons. If there were differences between MZ and DZ twinships, these, too, would have to be introduced into any type of analysis involving comparisons between MZ and DZ twinships (eg, the comparison of intratwinship correlations or heritability coefficients).

We have systematically studied the gestation, delivery, and first month of life using our newly devised questionnaire instrument (PDF) with 367 sets of twins. In addition, we have collected the same information on a subsample of singleton sibs of 44 pairs of twins.

The PDF instrument consists of three sections of questions concerning each of the areas of interest. The *pregnancy section* contains items such as length of gestation, various problems experienced during gestation, and various medications taken during pregnancy (what type, for how long).

The section on *delivery* elicits information on length of labor, difficulties during labor and delivery, each child's height and weight at birth, and any special problems experienced by the child at birth (eg, cyanosis, slow heart beat). The *first month of life* section is based on previous studies [Cohen et al, 1972] on the relation between an infant's global competence and later development, and can be used with singletons as well as twins. Questions cover a child's general health, bodily functions, attention, irritability, and vigor, and are scored on an operationally defined scale, ranging from no difficulties (optimal function) to major difficulties (poor functioning). One interpretation of the scores is to relate high scores with overall competence or maturity. Factor analysis of the PDF resulted in seven factors for pregnancy, three for delivery, and three for the first months of life.

Highlights of the interactions of the many effects of birth order, maternal age, children's sex, and children's zygosity were: Primigravidas had more problems with fluid retention, mothers of DZ males more than mothers of MZ; middle-class mothers had more problems with fluid retention; vaginal bleeding was greater as the mother's age increased if the twin pregnancy was her second one, if the twins were male, and, if she was in the higher socioeconomic class. Younger mothers, especially lower class, had more morning sickness than older women. Problems associated with pre-eclampsia were more common during the first pregnancies than succeeding ones, with mothers of DZ males having the least difficulty in this area.

The use of medication during pregnancy is of general concern in relation to birth defects, but is of special methodological concern in relation to the interpretation of twin data. Pharmacotherapy during gestation remains a poorly defined area of environmental influences on later development. In our study, mothers took an average of four drugs. The number of medications increased significantly with the age of the mother ($p < 0.001$), and concomitantly, with the number of previous pregnancies. Antiemetics, diuretics, and psychoactive medications were the most commonly used drugs, in addition to vitamins and iron preparations. Many questions are raised. For example, is one twin differentially affected by medications of different types? If so, is it the larger twin (who may be receiving a higher blood volume) or the smaller twin (who may be more immature)? What are the cumulative effects of age of mothers, social class, types of experienced difficulties, and medication?

At delivery, various factors suggested significant differences between groups of twins based on mother's obstetric history, zygosity, and sex, Monozygotic and dizygotic girl pairs had more cardiorespiratory problems than boys. Primigravidas had significantly longer labor than women with previous pregnancies, and less physically mature infants, $F = 5.12$, $p < 0.01$. The children in MZ pairs were born closer together than children in DZ twinships. The mean birthweight for first- and second-born twins was similar (2.4/kg), but there was significantly more variance for the secondborn (SD = 40) than for the firstborn (SD = 19). Monozygotic pairs were significantly less physically mature (birthweight, need for incubation, etc) than DZ pairs, but DZ pairs were generally less healthy, and less calm during the immediate newborn period. In general, secondborn males had more difficulties during the newborn period, with DZ males having more problems than MZ. Socioeconomic status seemed an important determinant in the infants' physical maturity, with the highest SES children having the best scores: $F = 4.76$, $p < 0.01$.

While the differences between MZ and DZ twinships, and between male and female children's prenatal and early newborn experiences, tended to be subtle, there were quite clear differences between the environmental experiences of twins and singletons on the pregnancy, delivery, and first month of life variables. The PDF information was obtained about the closest-in-age singleton sib of 44 sets of MZ and DZ twins. The twin pregnancies differed quite significantly from the gestations of their singleton sibs. Surprisingly, however, we found no significant differences in this small contrast sample in relation to variables associated with delivery. As would be expected, there were significant differences between twin A and B and the singleton sib on the First Month of Life scores with the single-born infant being more healthy and robust than either twin.

COMMENT

The assumption of equivalence of environmental experience is central to various uses of twins in psychological and developmental research. If MZ and DZ twins, and if male and female twins, all have significantly different prenatal and postnatal experiences, the explication of the mutual contributions of genetic and environmental factors becomes much more difficult. Complex, multivariate, and covariant models, rather than simpler MZ/DZ contrasts, would be demanded by interactional patterns involving sex, zygosity, parity, maternal age, and other variables.

The psychological experiences and the physiological experiences of MZ and DZ boy and girl twinships have been shown to differ from each other on various parameters; twins and singletons in critical areas (eg, exposure to medications). These environmental differences must be accounted for in models about genetic contributions and in models about the emergence of competence during the first months of life. Although this may make our work more difficult by the recognition of problems involved with the assumption of equivalence, the work is also made more interesting, and the complex interactions may suggest new hypotheses for future research.

REFERENCES

Bulmer MG (1970): "The Biology of Twinning in Man." London: Clarendon Press.

Cederlöf R, Friberg L, Jonsson E, Kaij L (1961): Studies on similarity diagnosis in twins with the aid of mailed questionnaires. Acta Genet 11:338–362.

Cohen DJ, Allen MG, Pollin W, Inoff G, Werner M, Dibble E (1972): Personality development in twins competence in the newborn and preschool periods. J Am Acad Child Psychiatry 11:625–644.

Cohen DJ, Dibble ED, Grawe JM, Pollin W (1973): Separating identical from fraternal twins. Arch Gen Psychiatry 29:465–469.

Cohen DJ, Dibble ED, Grawe JM, Pollin W (1975): Reliably separating identical from fraternal twins. Arch Gen Psychiatry 32:1371–1375.

Cohen DJ, Dibble ED, Grawe JM (1977a): Fathers' and mothers' perceptions of children's personality. Arch Gen Psychiatry 34:480–487.

Cohen DJ, Dibble ED, Grawe JM (1977b): Parental style. Arch Gen Psychiatry 34:445–455.

Corner GW (1955): The observed embryology of human single-ovum twins and other multiple births. Am J Obstet Gynecol 70:933–951.

Dibble ED, Grawe JM, Cohen DJ (1976): The association of child behavior with child rearing and family stress. Presented at the Annual Meeting of the American Academy of Child Psychiatry, October 1976, Toronto.

Galton F (1875): The history of twins as a criterion of the relative powers of nature and nurture. J Anthrop Inst 5:391–406.

Husen T (1959): "Psychological Twin Research." Stockholm: Almqvist and Wilksell.

Nichols RC, Bilbro WC (1966): The diagnosis of twin zygosity. Acta Genet 16:265–275.

Osborne RH, de George F (1955): Genetic basis of morphological variations: An evaluation and application of the twin study method. Cambridge, Massachusetts: Harvard University Press–Commonwealth Fund.

Siemens HW (1927): The diagnosis of identity in twins. J Hered 18:201–209.

Wilson RS (1970): Blood typing and twin zygosity. Hum Hered 20:30–56.

A Likelihood Ratio Test for Unequal Shared Environmental Variance in Twin Studies

Robert J Garrison, David L Demets, Richard R Fabsitz, and Manning Feinleib

INTRODUCTION

Several recent publications [Haseman et al, 1970; Christian et al, 1974; Hjortland, 1972] have suggested improvements for estimation and testing for genetic variation of quantitative data from twin studies. This report will present a new design and analysis which allows for a test of the important assumption of equal shared environmental variance in MZ and DZ twins. The approach requires stratifying the twin sample according to frequency of intrapair contact and testing for equality of shared environmental variance in the subgroups. Data from the National Heart, Lung, and Blood Institute (NHLBI) twin study will be analyzed by this method and recommendations as to interpretation and use of the method discussed.

METHODS

Adult male twins, aged 42–56 years, who were examined as part of the NHLBI twin study were asked, independently of their twin, "How often do you and your twin get together now?" Eighty-seven percent of the 514 twin pairs agreed that they "get together" either at least once a month (often) or less than once a month (seldom). These 217 MZ and 230 DZ twin pairs are those for whom results will be reported. For ease of notation, MZ and DZ twins will be designated M and D, while twins who report they "get together" often and seldom will be denoted O and S, respectively.

Quantitative measurements for the members of the i-th twin pair are assumed to be bivariate-normally distributed. Thus, the log likelihood function of a random

Twin Research: Psychology and Methodology, pages 253–259

sample of n independent twin pairs is given in Table I where the observations are written in terms of within (MSW) and among (MSA) mean squares. The likelihood function has one such set of terms specific for each of the four categories of twins, that is, MO, MS, DO, and DS. A joint likelihood function for all twins is written by substituting the number of twin pairs and the within- and among-pair mean squares for MO, MS, DO, and DS. In addition, the reparameterization of the likelihood function (in ρ and σ) is based on the model shown in Table I. If all effects are independent, then the parameterization shown in Table II for the four types of twins can be obtained. The joint log likelihood function is then written in terms of the seven parameters and the maximum value $L(x, \Theta_A)$ of the function is determined numerically using Maxlik [Kaplan et al, 1972].

The three null hypotheses to be tested are shown in Table III. These hypotheses are tested by maximizing the likelihood function under the appropriately restricted model. The value obtained, $L(x, \Theta_k)$, for each of the three null hypotheses is then tested against $L(x, \Theta_A)$, the value of the likelihood for the seven-parameter model, using the fact that for large samples $-2 \ln [L(x, \Theta_k)/L(x, \Theta_A)]$ is distributed approximately as chi-squared with degrees of freedom equal to the number of parameters by which the model is reduced under the null hypothesis.

RESULTS AND DISCUSSION

The particular variables presented in this paper were chosen purely as an aid to exposition, according to the results of significance tests for the various null hypotheses. Details of the measurement of these particular attributes are presented

TABLE I. Likelihood Function and Model for the Analysis of Twin Data

$$\ln L = -n \ln (2\pi\sigma^2 \sqrt{1-\rho^2}) - \frac{n \, MSW}{2\sigma^2 (1-\rho)} - \frac{(n-1) \, MSA}{2\sigma^2 (1+\rho)}$$

$Xij = \mu + Gij + Ei + Nij$

where

μ = mean population value

Gij = genetic deviation from mean in the j-th member of i-th pair

Ei = shared environmental deviation in the i-th pair

Nij = nonshared environmental deviation from mean in j-th member of i-th pair

TABLE II. Reparameterization of ρ and σ for MZ Often, MZ Seldom, DZ Often, and DZ Seldom Twin Pairs

For MO
$$\sigma^2(1-\rho) = \sigma^2_{NMO}$$
$$\sigma^2(1+\rho) = 2(\sigma^2_G + \sigma^2_{EO}) + \sigma^2_{NMO}$$
$$\sigma^2 = \sigma^2_G + \sigma^2_{EO} + \sigma^2_{NMO}$$

For MS
$$\sigma^2(1-\rho) = \sigma^2_{NMS}$$
$$\sigma^2(1+\rho) = 2(\sigma^2_G + \sigma^2_{ES}) + \sigma^2_{NMS}$$
$$\sigma^2 = \sigma^2_G + \sigma^2_{ES} + \sigma^2_{NMS}$$

For DO
$$\sigma^2(1-\rho) = 1/2\,\sigma^2_G + \sigma^2_{NDO}$$
$$\sigma^2(1+\rho) = 3/2\,\sigma^2_G + 2\sigma^2_{EO} + \sigma^2_{NDO}$$
$$\sigma^2 = \sigma^2_G + \sigma^2_{EO} + \sigma^2_{NDO}$$

For DS
$$\sigma^2(1-\rho) = 1/2\,\sigma^2_G + \sigma^2_{NDS}$$
$$\sigma^2(1+\rho) = 3/2\,\sigma^2_G + 2\sigma^2_{ES} + \sigma^2_{NS}$$
$$\sigma^2 = \sigma^2_G + \sigma^2_{ES} + \sigma^2_{NDS}$$

TABLE III. Null Hypotheses of Interest

1. $\sigma^2_{NMO} = \sigma^2_{NMS} = \sigma^2_{NDO} = \sigma^2_{NDS}$
2. $\sigma^2_{EO} = \sigma^2_{ES}$
3. $\sigma^2_G = 0$

elsewhere [Feinleib et al, 1977]. For cholesterol carried on the low-density lipoprotein (LDL) all three of the null hypotheses are rejected in Table IV. Null hypothesis 1 is analogous to the F' test proposed by Haseman and Elston [1970] for equality of MZ and DZ variances. The result for LDL strongly suggests heterogeneity of variance across the four twin groups, much of it apparently due to the difference between MZ and DZ twins as previously noted in these data (Feinleib et al, 1977]. Null hypothesis 2 is also rejected at a very high level of significance.

TABLE IV. Observations and Results of Likelihood Ratio Tests for LDL Cholesterol

	Often		Seldom	
	MZ	DZ	MZ	DZ
Number	154	107	60	116
$\overline{X}$	144.0	139.0	145.7	145.8
MSW	402.8	872.0	358.9	893.6
MSA	2,127.4	2,133.3	1,522.7	1,804.8

Null hypothesis	df	χ^2	P
$\sigma^2_{NMO} = \sigma^2_{NMS} = \sigma^2_{NDO} = \sigma^2_{NDS}$	3	117.70	<0.001
$\sigma^2_{EO} = \sigma^2_{ES}$	1	14.52	<0.001
$\sigma^2_G = 0$	1	5.32	0.02

This test indicates that twins who see each other often have greater shared environmental variation for LDL cholesterol. It is important to notice in Table IV that MZ twins "get together" considerably more often than do DZ twins. This finding, together with rejection of hypothesis 2, indicates that MZ twins have more similar LDL cholesterol levels than do DZ twins for reasons other than their relative genetic similarity. Null hypothesis 3 is analogous to the likelihood ratio test for genetic variance proposed by Hjortland [1972]. For LDL cholesterol the P value for null hypothesis 3 is comparable to that which has been reported previously (P = 0.06) for the F' test using data on all 514 twin pairs [Feinleib et al, 1977].

For alkaline phosphatase skewness in the distribution of observations was markedly reduced by considering the log of each measurement ($\times$ 100). As shown in Table V, there is no heterogeneity of nonshared environmental effects but, again, considerable evidence for unequal shared environmental variance for O and S twins. In addition, there is highly significant genetic variation. Comparison of the results for LDL and alkaline phosphatase points out the possible different interpretations of data for which hypothesis 2 is rejected. On one hand, it is not difficult to speculate that, if significantly different shared environmental variance can be demonstrated using this particular stratification scheme, there must be considerable confounding of genetic variance and shared environmental variance within the sample, and it is doubtful that true genetic variance could ever be

TABLE V. Observations and Results of Likelihood Ratio Tests for Alkaline Phosphatase

	Often		Seldom	
	MZ	DZ	MZ	DZ
Number	153	110	60	120
$\bar{X}$	170.8	171.8	172.3	172.0
MSW	64.7	131.7	54.0	95.4
MSA	540.2	530.9	439.2	384.8

Null hypothesis	df	χ^2	P
$\sigma^2_{NMO} = \sigma^2_{NMS} = \sigma^2_{NDO} = \sigma^2_{NDS}$	3	3.83	NS
$\sigma^2_{EO} = \sigma^2_{ES}$	1	18.97	<0.001
$\sigma^2_G = 0$	1	12.91	<0.001

estimated for the particular variable using a twin study. This rather conservative approach might be favored for a variable showing less genetic variation, such as LDL. On the other hand, it is certainly possible that both genetic variation and shared environmental variation are present for a particular variable. In such a case one would speculate that the stratification reduces the confounding of genetic and shared environmental variation. It might be appropriate to attach such an interpretation to alkaline phosphatase in view of the highly significant test for genetic variation.

The interpretation of the test for genetic variance for systolic blood pressure (Table VI) is uncomplicated since null hypothesis 2 is not rejected. However, the staunch critic of twin studies can argue that acceptance of null hypothesis 2 in this case does not validate the twin analysis; it shows only that this particular stratification scheme fails to uncover alleged differences in shared environment in MZ and DZ twins.

The confounding of genetic variance and shared environmental variance is a major potential flaw in the twin method. The design and analysis presented here attempts to detect variables for which such confounding could lead to overestimation of genetic variance. Obviously, there may be better criteria on which to stratify twin samples. The present scheme has no clear implications as to effects occurring early in life. However, pursuing this type of design and analysis should increase confidence in estimates of genetic variance from twin studies.

TABLE VI. Observations and Results of Likelihood Ratio Tests for Systolic Blood Pressure

	Often		Seldom	
	MZ	DZ	MZ	DZ
Number	156	110	61	120
$\overline{X}$	129.6	127.6	130.6	127.7
MSW	146.1	184.9	151.7	212.7
MSA	520.0	365.0	633.0	327.9

Null hypothesis	df	χ^2	P
$\sigma^2_{NMO} = \sigma^2_{NMS} = \sigma^2_{NDO} = \sigma^2_{NDS}$	3	5.85	NS
$\sigma^2_{EO} = \sigma^2_{ES}$	1	0.04	NS
$\sigma^2_{G} = 0$	1	25.60	<0.001

There is another important implication of the results from this design and analysis. For a variable such as LDL cholesterol which exhibits significantly greater shared environmental variance for twins who "get together" often, there is an indication that factors associated with frequency of contact influence LDL variation. For a variable such as LDL cholesterol, which in epidemiologic studies has virtually defied "prediction," such findings are of considerable interest.

SUMMARY

The results of this study of adult male twins indicate that, for LDL cholesterol and alkaline phosphatase, there is evidence that twins who "get together" often exhibit greater shared environmental variance. Since in this study such twins are more likely to be MZ, conclusions about genetic variance for LDL cholesterol and alkaline phosphatase must be tempered or totally discarded. It is concluded that this design, while strengthening the twin method, does not provide absolute assurance that confounding of shared environmental variance and genetic variance does not occur.

Contents to Part C: Clinical Studies

Index